# Fuel Your Potential, Embrace Smart Eating Habits!



*Disclaimer: The information provided in this book is for educational purposes only and is not intended as medical advice. Always consult with a qualified healthcare professional before making any changes to your diet or lifestyle. The author and publisher of this book are not responsible for any adverse effects or consequences resulting from the use of the information provided herein.*

Dear Reader,

Thank you so much for your purchase of "Smart Eating Habits: Fuel your Potential, Embrace Smart Eating Habits" Your support means the world to us, and we hope this book will provide you with valuable insights and practical guidance on your journey to optimal health.

I have poured my heart into creating this book, and I genuinely hope it has exceeded your expectations. I would love to hear your thoughts and experiences with the content.

Take the time to read the book and understand its content and message and once done, if you enjoyed reading "Smart Eating Habits," I kindly invite you to leave a review on the platform where you made your purchase. Your feedback not only helps improve any future content but also assists other readers in discovering the benefits of this book.

Your review will be a powerful testament to the impact of smart eating habits on our lives. It's through your support and feedback that I can continue to create more amazing content to empower and inspire others to prioritize their well-being.

Once again, thank you for joining us on this journey. I am grateful to have you as part of our community, and I look forward to providing you with even more valuable resources and insights in the future.

With warmest regards,

Steven Clinch

www.smarteatinghabits.com

# Table of Contents

# Introduction

In today's fast-paced world, people are busier than ever and often find it difficult to prioritize healthy eating habits. However, eating a balanced diet full of nutrient-rich foods is essential for maintaining optimal physical and mental health. The purpose of this e-book, titled "Smart Eating Habits," is to provide readers with the knowledge and tools necessary to make informed decisions about their food choices and develop healthy eating habits.

Chapter One, "Why Eat Healthy?" will explore the many benefits of eating a healthy diet, including weight management, disease prevention, improved energy levels, and better mental health. It will also discuss the consequences of a poor diet, such as obesity, chronic illness, and decreased cognitive function.

Chapter Two, "Understanding Your Relationship with Food," will delve into the psychological and emotional aspects of eating, including how our past experiences and social influences shape our food choices. It will also explore the concept of mindful eating and how it can help us develop a healthier relationship with food.

Chapter Three, "How Food Can Be Your Medicine," will explore the healing properties of certain foods and how they can be used to treat and prevent illness. It will also discuss the importance of a varied and balanced diet in promoting overall health and wellness.

Chapter Four, "The Dangers of Diet Trends," will examine the risks and potential benefits of popular diet trends, such as keto, paleo, and veganism. It will also provide guidance on how to choose a diet plan that is safe, sustainable, and tailored to your individual needs.

Chapter Five, "The Health Benefits of Eating Fruits," will explore the many health benefits of incorporating fruits into your diet, including their rich antioxidant content, fiber, and essential vitamins and minerals.

Chapter Six, "The Health Benefits of Eating Vegetables," will delve into the many health benefits of incorporating vegetables into your diet, including their anti-inflammatory properties, fiber content, and vitamin and mineral density.

Chapter Seven, "The Best Meat to Eat for Healthy Living," will examine the nutritional properties of various types of meat and provide guidance on choosing the healthiest options.

Chapter Eight, "The Dangers of Processed Foods," will explore the potential health risks associated with consuming processed foods and provide guidance on how to minimize their intake.

Chapter Nine, "Dangers of Food Additives," will examine the various food additives commonly used in processed foods and their potential risks and health effects.

Chapter Ten, "Bringing It All Together with Meal Planning," will provide practical tips and guidance on how to plan and prepare healthy meals that are both satisfying and nutritious.

In conclusion, "Smart Eating Habits" aims to empower readers with the knowledge and tools necessary to make informed decisions about their food choices and develop healthy eating habits that will promote optimal physical and mental health.

By adopting these habits, readers can take control of their health and well-being and enjoy the many benefits of a balanced, nutrient-rich diet.

# Chapter 1: The Importance of a Healthy Diet

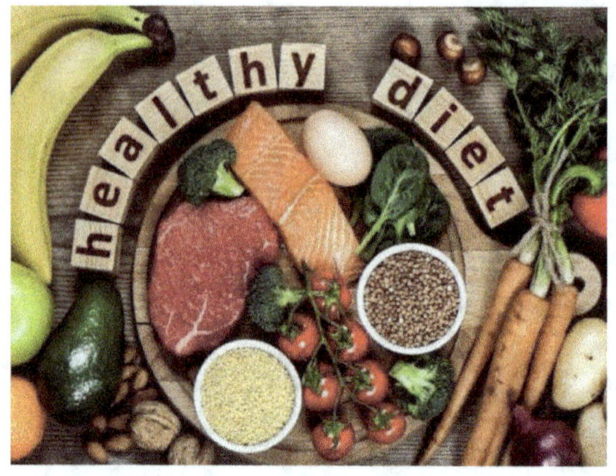


A healthy diet is essential for good health and well-being. It provides the body with the necessary nutrients to function optimally and to prevent chronic diseases.

A healthy diet is not just about consuming the right number of calories but also involves eating a variety of foods that provide essential nutrients, including vitamins, minerals, protein, fiber, and healthy fats.

## What is a Healthy Diet?

A healthy diet is one that provides all the necessary nutrients that the body needs to function optimally. It should contain a variety of whole, unprocessed foods from different food groups, such as fruits, vegetables, whole grains, lean protein, and healthy fats. It should also limit the intake of processed and sugary foods, saturated and trans fats, and excessive amounts of salt.

A healthy diet should be balanced, which means that it should provide adequate amounts of macronutrients (carbohydrates, protein, and fat) as well as micronutrients (vitamins and minerals). It should also be sustainable and enjoyable, which means that it should be a long-term lifestyle rather than a short-term diet.

Focusing on a variety of colorful fruits and vegetables is important for a healthy diet. These foods are rich in vitamins, minerals, fiber, and phytochemicals, which all play important roles in maintaining optimal health. Whole grains such as brown rice, whole wheat bread, and quinoa are also important for providing fiber and other essential nutrients.

Lean protein sources such as chicken, fish, beans, and legumes should also be part of a healthy diet.

They provide essential amino acids that the body needs to build and repair tissues, as well as supporting immune function, and providing the needed energy.

## Essential Nutrients in a Healthy Diet

A healthy diet should include essential nutrients that are necessary for proper bodily functions. These nutrients include carbohydrates, proteins, fats, vitamins, and minerals. Carbohydrates provide the body with energy, while proteins are necessary for building and repairing tissues. Fats are important for energy production, hormone regulation, and brain function.

Vitamins and minerals are also important in a healthy diet. Vitamins such as vitamin C, vitamin A, and vitamin D are important for immune function, vision, and bone health, respectively. Minerals such as calcium, iron, and zinc are also essential for proper bodily functions.

# Balanced Eating Patterns and Portion Control

Maintaining a balanced eating pattern and portion control are key components of a healthy diet. A balanced eating pattern involves consuming a variety of foods from different food groups in the right proportions. This ensures that the body receives all the necessary nutrients that it needs to function optimally.

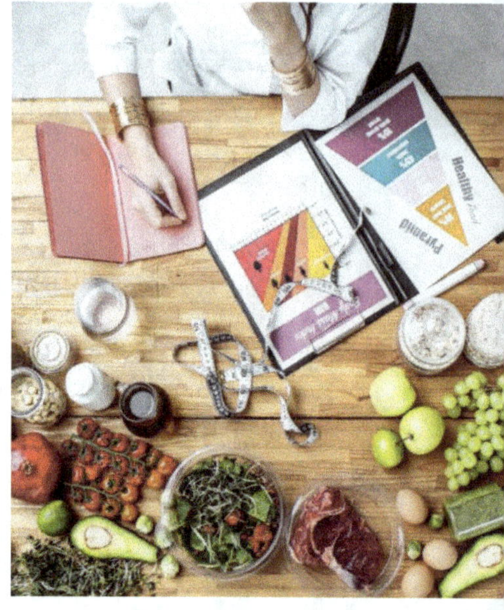

Portion control is also important to ensure that the body receives the right amount of energy it needs. Consuming too much food can lead to weight gain, while consuming too little food can lead to malnutrition.

Balancing calorie intake with physical activity is also essential for maintaining a healthy weight.

To achieve balanced eating patterns and portion control, it is important to practice mindful eating. This involves paying attention to hunger and fullness cues, eating slowly, and savoring each bite. Planning meals ahead of time and controlling portion sizes can also be helpful strategies.

# The various risks associated with an unhealthy diet.

An unhealthy diet can increase the risk of various health problems, including obesity, heart disease, stroke, diabetes, and certain types of cancer. Poor nutrition, including a diet high in saturated and trans fats, sugar, and salt, can lead to weight gain, which is a risk factor for many chronic diseases.

**Obesity** is one of the most significant risks associated with an unhealthy diet. When we consume more calories than our body needs, we store the excess energy as fat, leading to weight gain. Obesity is linked to many health problems, including heart disease, stroke, diabetes, and certain types of cancer. Obesity can also lead to physical limitations, decreased quality of life, and reduced life expectancy.

**Heart disease and stroke** are two other risks associated with an unhealthy diet. A diet high in saturated and trans fats, cholesterol, and salt can increase blood pressure and blood cholesterol levels, leading to the accumulation of plaque in the arteries. This can eventually lead to heart disease and stroke, which are among the leading causes of death in the United States.

**Diabetes** is also a risk associated with an unhealthy diet. A diet high in sugar and refined carbohydrates can lead to insulin resistance, which can eventually lead to type 2 diabetes. Diabetes can lead to a host of complications, including blindness, kidney disease, nerve damage, and amputations.

Certain types of **cancer** are also linked to an unhealthy diet. A diet high in processed foods, red meat, and saturated fat has been linked to an increased risk of colorectal cancer. Similarly, a diet high in saturated fat has been linked to an increased risk of breast cancer.

Apart from these risks, an unhealthy diet can also lead to poor mental health. A diet high in sugar, refined carbohydrates, and unhealthy fats has been linked to depression, anxiety, and other mental health problems. In contrast, a healthy diet rich in whole grains, fruits, vegetables, and lean protein have been linked to better mental health.

The risks associated with an unhealthy diet are not limited to physical health problems. Poor nutrition can also affect **cognitive function**, memory, and mood. A diet high in sugar, unhealthy fats, and processed foods has been linked to cognitive decline, memory problems, and increased risk of dementia.

## Common myths and misconceptions surrounding diet and nutrition.

There are many myths and misconceptions about diet and nutrition that can lead people down the wrong path. Here are some of the most common myths and misconceptions:

1.  Fad diets are necessary for weight loss: Many people believe that fad diets are the only way to lose weight quickly. However, these diets are often unhealthy and can lead to long-term health problems. A healthy and sustainable approach to weight loss is through a balanced and nutritious diet combined with regular exercise.

2. Carbohydrates are bad for you: Carbohydrates are an important source of energy for the body and cutting them out completely can lead to a lack of energy and other health problems. It is important to choose healthy sources of carbohydrates, such as whole grains, fruits, and vegetables.

3. All fats are bad for you: While it is true that some types of fats can be harmful in large amounts, not all fats are created equal. Healthy fats, such as those found in nuts, seeds, and fatty fish, are essential for a healthy diet and can help to lower the risk of heart disease and other health problems.

4. Expensive supplements are necessary for good health: While some supplements may be beneficial for certain health conditions, most people can get all the nutrients they need from a balanced diet. It is important to consult a healthcare professional before taking any supplements, as some can interact with medications or have harmful side effects.

5. Eating healthy is expensive: While it is true that some healthy foods can be more expensive than processed or junk foods, it is possible to eat a healthy diet on a budget. Choosing seasonal produce, buying in bulk, and cooking at home can all help to save money while still eating a nutritious diet.

6. Skipping meals is a good way to lose weight: Skipping meals can actually be harmful to your health and can lead to overeating later on. It is important to eat regular meals and snacks throughout the day to maintain a healthy weight and provide the body with the nutrients it needs.

By understanding and dispelling these myths and misconceptions, individuals can make informed choices about their diet and nutrition and lead a healthier and happier life.

# Chapter 2: Mindful Eating: Understanding Your Relationship with Food

## What is Mindful Eating?

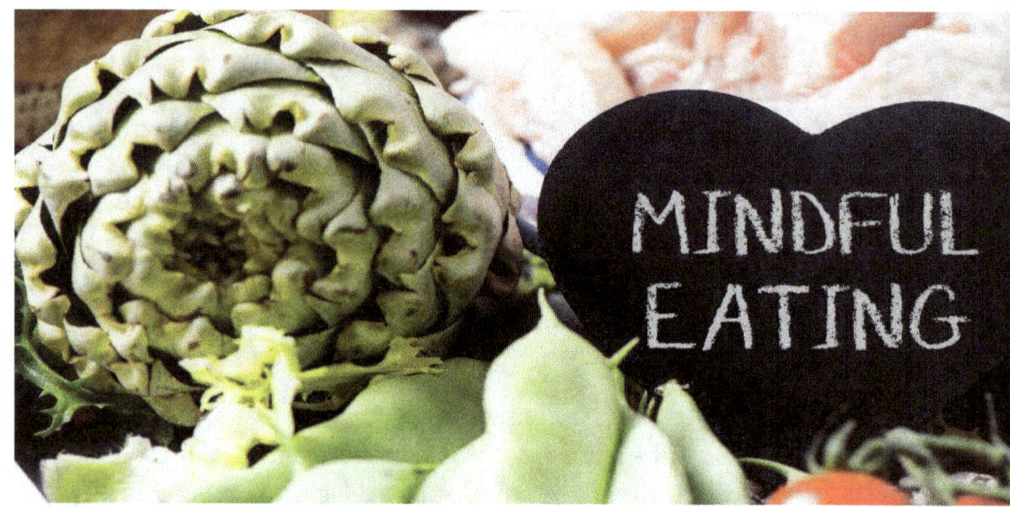


Mindful eating is a practice of being present and fully engaged while eating. It involves paying attention to the sensory experiences of food, such as its taste, texture, and aroma, and being aware of one's feelings and thoughts around food.

Mindful eating is different from mindless eating, which is characterized by consuming food without awareness or attention, often while engaged in other activities such as watching TV or scrolling through social media. Unlike mindless eating, mindful eating focuses on the experience of eating and aims to cultivate a deeper connection with food and the body.

# The benefits of practicing mindful eating.

The benefits of practicing mindful eating are numerous and wide-ranging. One of the key benefits is improved digestion. When we practice mindful eating, we are more aware of our body's hunger and fullness cues, which allows us to eat until we are satisfied without overeating.

This can lead to better digestion, as our body is better able to process and utilize the nutrients from the food we consume. Additionally, mindful eating can help reduce digestive discomfort and bloating, as we become more aware of how different foods affect our body.

Another benefit of mindful eating is better food choices. When we are present and engaged with the experience of eating, we are more likely to make intentional choices about what we eat. This can lead to a greater appreciation for healthy, nourishing foods and a reduction in the consumption of processed junk foods.

Mindful eating can also help us develop a deeper understanding of our personal food preferences and cravings, allowing us to make choices that align with our individual needs and values.

In addition to these benefits, practicing mindful eating can also help promote mindful living more generally. By cultivating a sense of presence and awareness around food, we may become more attuned to our thoughts, feelings, and bodily sensations in other areas of life as well. This can lead to a greater sense of self-awareness and overall well-being.

Overall, the benefits of practicing mindful eating are numerous and wide-ranging.

By fostering a deeper connection with food and the body, mindful eating can lead to improved digestion, better food choices, reduced stress levels, and a more positive relationship with eating and the self.

# The Importance of Listening to Your Body

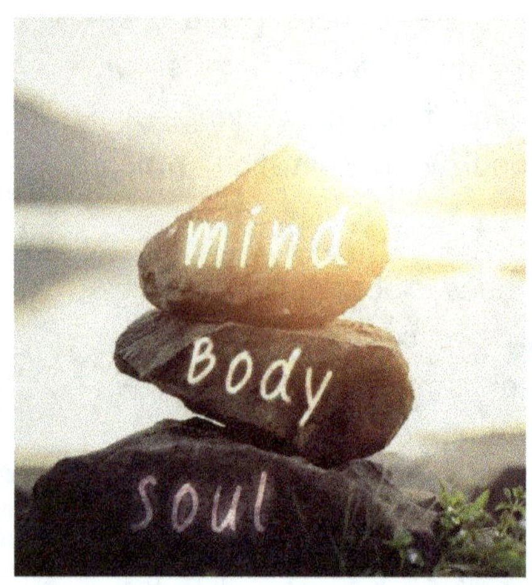


Listening to your body is an essential part of maintaining a healthy lifestyle. Your body is incredibly intelligent and is constantly giving you signals about what it needs.

Unfortunately, in our busy lives, we often ignore these signals and make poor choices that can lead to health problems. However, by learning to tune in to your body's needs and listening to its signals, you can improve your health and well-being.

One of the most important things you can do to listen to your body is to pay attention to hunger and fullness cues. When you eat, it's essential to eat until you're satisfied, not until you're stuffed.

This helps prevent overeating, which can lead to weight gain and other health issues. Conversely, if you don't eat enough, your body will tell you by sending hunger signals, which can lead to low energy and other problems.

Another critical aspect of listening to your body is being aware of how different foods affect you. Certain foods may cause digestive issues, while others can lead to inflammation or allergic reactions.

 By paying attention to how your body feels after you eat, you can identify which foods work well for you and which ones don't.

In addition to physical cues, your body also sends emotional signals that are important to pay attention to.

For example, stress and anxiety can manifest in physical symptoms such as headaches, muscle tension, and fatigue.

By listening to these signals, you can identify the root cause of your stress and take steps to manage it, such as meditation or exercise.

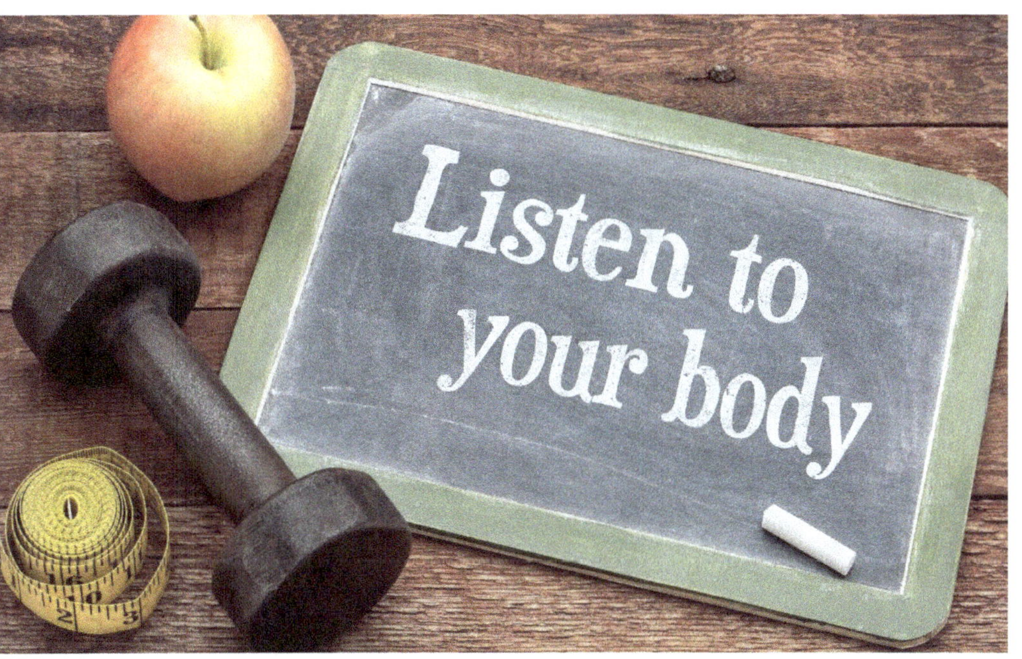

# Building a Healthy Relationship with Food

Building a healthy relationship with food is an important aspect of maintaining a healthy diet and overall well-being. It involves changing one's mindset about food and understanding that it is not just about nourishment, but also about enjoyment and satisfaction.

Here are some tips for building a healthy relationship with food:

1.  **Eat mindfully**: As discussed in the previous pages, mindful eating is about paying attention to your body's hunger and fullness cues and being present in the moment while eating. It also involves eating slowly and savoring the flavors and textures of your food.

2.  **Practice intuitive eating**: Intuitive eating is about trusting your body to tell you what and how much to eat. It involves listening to your hunger and fullness cues, as well as your cravings, and making choices that satisfy your body's needs.

3.  **Avoid restrictive diets**: Restrictive diets can lead to a negative relationship with food, as they often involve depriving yourself of certain foods or food groups. Instead of focusing on restriction, try to focus on incorporating a variety of whole, nutrient-dense foods into your diet.

4.  **Be kind to yourself**: It's important to treat yourself with compassion and understanding when it comes to food. Avoid labeling foods as "good" or "bad," and try not to beat yourself up overindulgences or slip-ups.

5.  **Cook and prepare your own meals**: Cooking your own meals allows you to have control over the ingredients and the way your food is prepared. It can also be a fun and creative way to experiment with different flavors and cuisines.

6.  **Practice gratitude**: Taking the time to appreciate and be thankful for the food on your plate can help foster a positive

relationship with food. Try to focus on the nourishment and enjoyment that food provides, rather than just the calories or nutritional content.


By building a healthy relationship with food, you can not only improve your physical health, but also your mental and emotional well-being.

# Chapter 3: The Healing Power of Food

The concept of "food as medicine" refers to the idea that the food we eat can have a powerful impact on our health and well-being. By choosing nutrient-dense foods and incorporating them into our diets on a regular basis, we can potentially prevent and even treat a variety of health conditions.

This concept is supported by the idea that food contains various bioactive compounds that can have therapeutic effects on the body.

The approach of using food as medicine emphasizes the importance of whole, minimally processed foods and encourages individuals to focus on eating a balanced, varied diet that includes plenty of fruits, vegetables, whole grains, lean protein, and healthy fats.

## Anti-Inflammatory Foods

Inflammation is a natural response of the body to injury, infection, or irritation. It is a defense mechanism designed to protect the body by removing harmful stimuli and initiating the healing process. However, chronic inflammation can lead to a host of negative effects on the body, including increased risk of chronic diseases such as heart disease, diabetes, and cancer.

Inflammation can also exacerbate symptoms of existing conditions such as arthritis and asthma.

Anti-inflammatory foods are those that can help reduce inflammation in the body. They typically contain high levels of antioxidants, vitamins, and minerals that can help combat free radicals, reduce oxidative stress, and boost the immune system.

Some common examples of anti-inflammatory foods include:

- **Berries**: Berries are high in antioxidants, which can help protect the body against inflammation and oxidative stress. Blueberries, strawberries, raspberries, and blackberries are all excellent sources of anti-inflammatory compounds.

- **Leafy greens**: Leafy greens such as spinach, kale, and collard greens are rich in vitamins, minerals, and antioxidants that can help reduce inflammation in the body.

- **Fatty fish**: Fatty fish such as salmon, mackerel, and tuna are high in omega-3 fatty acids, which have been shown to have potent anti-inflammatory effects.

- **Nuts and seeds**: Nuts and seeds are high in healthy fats, fiber, and antioxidants, all of which can help reduce inflammation in the body. Examples include almonds, walnuts, chia seeds, and flaxseeds.

- **Turmeric**: Turmeric is a spice that contains a compound called curcumin, which has potent anti-inflammatory effects. It has been shown to be effective in reducing inflammation in conditions such as arthritis, and may also have benefits for heart health and brain function.

Incorporating anti-inflammatory foods into your diet can have several health benefits. In addition to reducing inflammation in the body, these foods may also help improve digestion, boost immune function, and reduce the risk of chronic diseases.

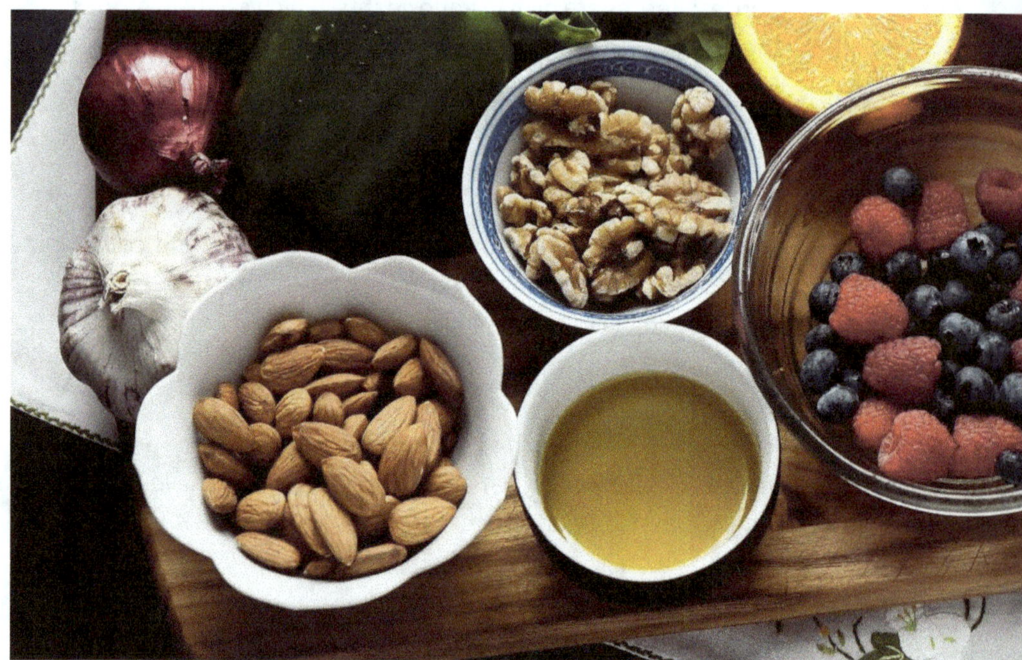

However, it's important to remember that no single food can cure or prevent disease, and that a healthy diet should be balanced and varied.

# Immune-Boosting Foods

The immune system is a complex network of cells, tissues, and organs that work together to protect the body against harmful microorganisms and foreign substances. A strong immune system is essential for overall health and wellbeing. It can prevent infections, reduce the risk of chronic diseases, and improve recovery from illness. Here are some of the reasons why having a strong immune system is important:

Fighting infections: The immune system is responsible for identifying and neutralizing viruses, bacteria, and other harmful pathogens that can cause infections.

Preventing chronic diseases: Chronic inflammation can weaken the immune system and increase the risk of chronic diseases such as heart disease, diabetes, and cancer.

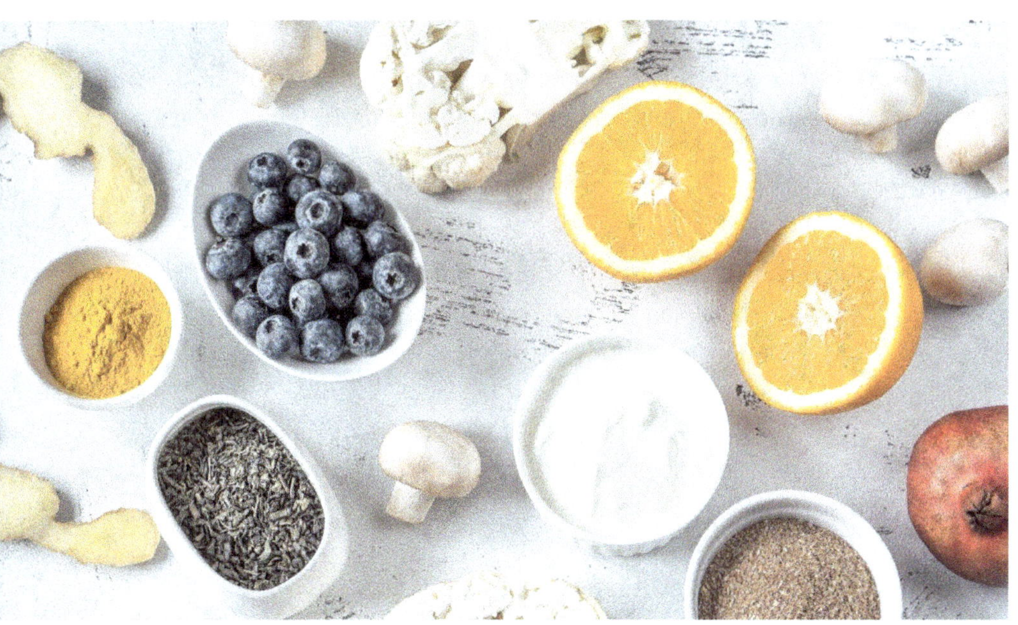

Improving recovery: A strong immune system can help the body recover more quickly from illness or injury.

There are many foods that can help boost the immune system. These foods contain nutrients such as vitamins A, C, and E, as well as zinc, selenium, and probiotics. Here are some examples of immune-boosting foods and their health benefits:

- **Citrus fruits**: Citrus fruits such as oranges, lemons, and grapefruits are high in vitamin C, which helps boost the immune system by increasing the production of white blood cells.

- **Berries**: Berries are rich in antioxidants, which can help reduce inflammation and improve immune function.

- **Leafy greens**: Leafy greens such as spinach and kale are high in vitamins A and C, as well as other antioxidants and nutrients that can help strengthen the immune system.

- **Garlic**: Garlic has anti-inflammatory and antimicrobial properties that can help boost the immune system and fight infections.

- **Ginger**: Ginger has anti-inflammatory and antioxidant properties that can help improve immune function and reduce inflammation in the body.

- **Yogurt**: Yogurt is rich in probiotics, which are beneficial bacteria that can help improve gut health and boost the immune system.

- **Nuts and seeds**: Nuts and seeds such as almonds, walnuts, and sunflower seeds are rich in vitamin E and other nutrients that can help boost the immune system.

# Foods for Brain Health

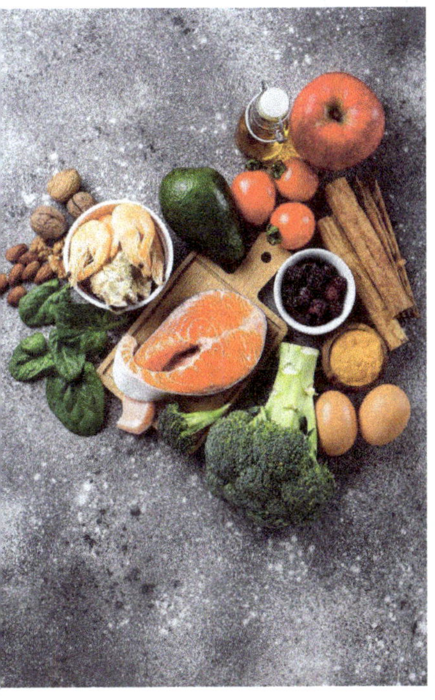

The human brain is the control center of the body, responsible for regulating various bodily functions, thoughts, and emotions. Therefore, it is crucial to maintain good brain health to ensure optimal cognitive functioning and mental well-being.

Research has shown that a healthy diet can significantly impact brain health and reduce the risk of cognitive decline and neurological disorders such as Alzheimer's disease and dementia.

A diet rich in nutrients such as omega-3 fatty acids, antioxidants, and B-vitamins can help promote brain function and support memory, concentration, and mood.

Here are some of the best brain-healthy foods to include in your diet:

- **Fatty fish**: Fish such as salmon, mackerel, and sardines are rich in omega-3 fatty acids, which play a vital role in brain health. Omega-3 fatty acids have been shown to improve brain function, reduce inflammation, and decrease the risk of cognitive decline.

- **Berries**: Berries such as blueberries, strawberries, and blackberries are packed with antioxidants that can help protect the brain from oxidative stress and inflammation. These antioxidants can help improve brain function and reduce the risk of age-related cognitive decline.

- **Nuts and seeds**: Nuts and seeds such as almonds, walnuts, chia seeds, and flaxseeds are excellent sources of vitamin E, which can help protect the brain from oxidative damage. They also contain healthy fats and other nutrients that can support brain function and improve memory and concentration.

- **Dark chocolate**: Dark chocolate contains flavonoids, which have been shown to improve blood flow to the brain and enhance cognitive function. It also contains caffeine and theobromine, which can improve mood and concentration.

- **Leafy greens**: Leafy greens such as spinach, kale, and collard greens are rich in nutrients such as folate, vitamin K, and antioxidants that can help protect the brain and reduce the risk of cognitive decline.

- **Whole grains**: Whole grains such as brown rice, quinoa, and whole-wheat bread are excellent sources of B-vitamins, which can help support brain function and reduce the risk of cognitive decline.

- **Turmeric**: Turmeric contains curcumin, a compound with powerful anti-inflammatory properties. It has been shown to improve brain function and reduce the risk of cognitive decline.

By incorporating these brain-healthy foods into your diet, you can help support brain function, improve memory, concentration, and mood, and reduce the risk of cognitive decline and neurological disorders.

# Foods for Heart Health

Heart health is a crucial aspect of overall health and well-being. The heart is responsible for pumping blood and supplying oxygen and nutrients to the body's organs and tissues. Maintaining a healthy heart is essential for preventing heart disease, which can lead to serious health issues such as heart attacks, strokes, and heart failure.

List of Heart-Healthy Foods and Their Health Benefits:

- **Berries**: Berries are rich in antioxidants, which can help protect the heart from damage caused by free radicals. They are also high in fiber, which can help lower cholesterol levels and reduce the risk of heart disease.

- **Leafy Green Vegetables**: Leafy greens like spinach, kale, and collard greens are high in vitamins, minerals, and antioxidants that can help reduce inflammation and improve heart health.

- **Fatty Fish**: Fatty fish like salmon, tuna, and mackerel are rich in omega-3 fatty acids, which can help reduce inflammation, lower triglyceride levels, and improve heart health.

- **Nuts**: Nuts like almonds, walnuts, and pistachios are high in healthy fats, fiber, and antioxidants, which can help reduce inflammation and improve heart health.

- **Whole Grains**: Whole grains like oats, quinoa, and brown rice are high in fiber and can help lower cholesterol levels, reduce the risk of heart disease, and improve overall heart health.

- **Legumes**: Legumes like chickpeas, lentils, and beans are high in fiber, protein, and other nutrients that can help lower cholesterol levels, reduce inflammation, and improve heart health.

- **Tomatoes**: Tomatoes are rich in lycopene, an antioxidant that can help protect the heart from damage caused by free radicals. They are also high in potassium, which can help lower blood pressure and improve heart health.

- **Dark Chocolate**: Dark chocolate is rich in flavonoids, which can help reduce inflammation, improve circulation, and lower blood pressure, all of which can help improve heart health.

By incorporating these heart-healthy foods into your diet, you can help improve your heart health and reduce the risk of heart disease.

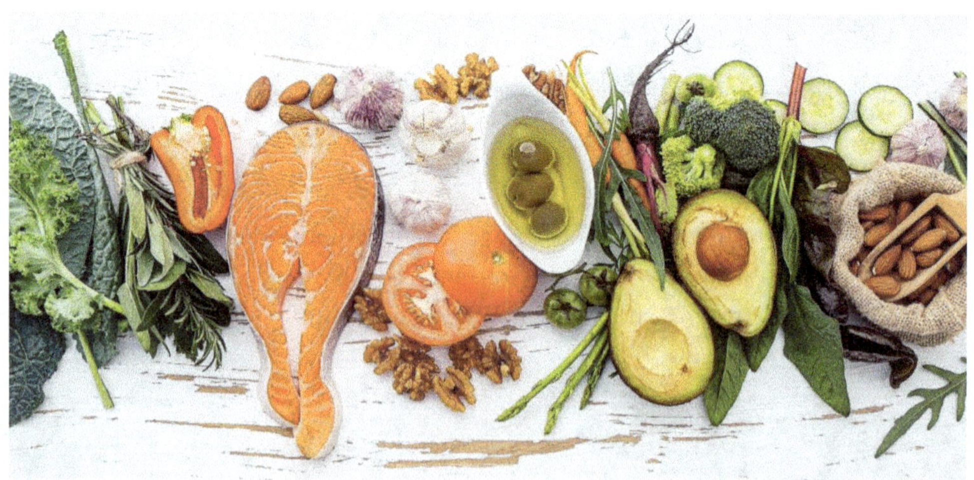

# Digestive Health Foods

Digestive health is vital for overall well-being, as it ensures that the body absorbs essential nutrients and gets rid of waste effectively. A healthy digestive system also supports a robust immune system and helps prevent various health issues, such as constipation, diarrhea, and irritable bowel syndrome (IBS).

The importance of digestive health is often underestimated, but it can have a significant impact on overall health. Digestive problems can lead to malnutrition, dehydration, and a weakened immune system, making it easier to get sick. It is essential to include foods in your diet that can support and promote digestive health.

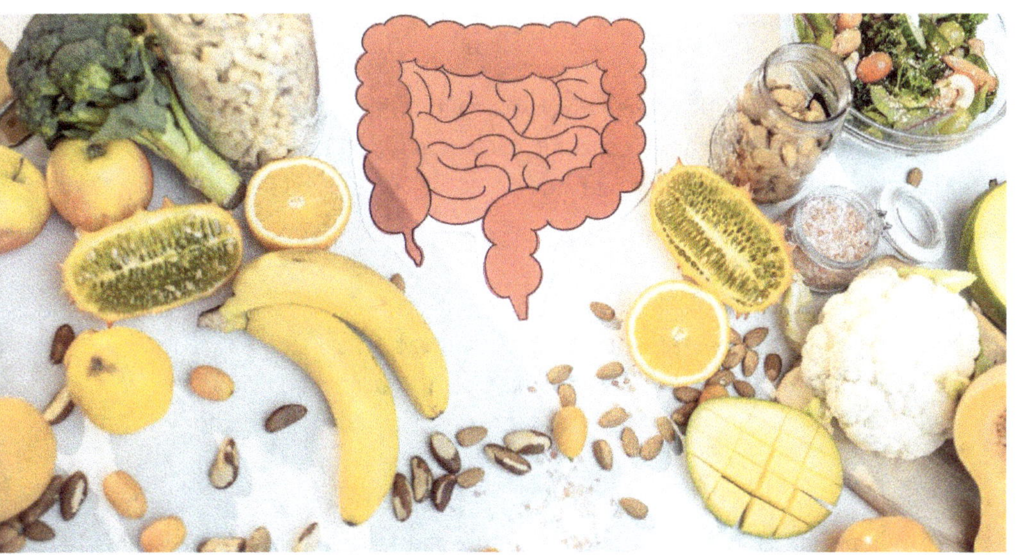

**Foods that are high in fiber** are particularly beneficial for digestive health. Fiber helps to move waste through the digestive system and can prevent constipation. It also feeds the beneficial bacteria in the gut, which helps to maintain a healthy balance of microorganisms.

**Probiotics** are also crucial for digestive health. They are live microorganisms that can help to balance the gut flora and support healthy digestion. Some probiotic-rich foods include yogurt, kefir, kimchi, sauerkraut, and other fermented foods.

**Antioxidant-rich foods**, such as fruits and vegetables, can also support digestive health. Antioxidants can help to reduce inflammation in the gut and prevent damage to the cells lining the digestive tract.

**Omega-3 fatty acids**, found in foods like fatty fish and flaxseed, can also support digestive health. They can reduce inflammation in the gut and help to maintain the integrity of the gut lining.

Incorporating **prebiotic foods**, which are high in fiber and can help to feed the beneficial bacteria in the gut, can also support digestive health. Some prebiotic-rich foods include onions, garlic, bananas, and asparagus.

**Drinking plenty of water** and staying hydrated is also essential for digestive health. Water helps to soften stools and prevent constipation, while also supporting the transport of nutrients throughout the body.

Overall, a diet rich in fiber, probiotics, antioxidants, omega-3 fatty acids, and prebiotics can help to promote digestive health and prevent various digestive problems. It is also crucial to stay hydrated and limit the intake of processed foods, which can be detrimental to digestive health.

# Chapter 4: The Truth About Popular Diet Trend

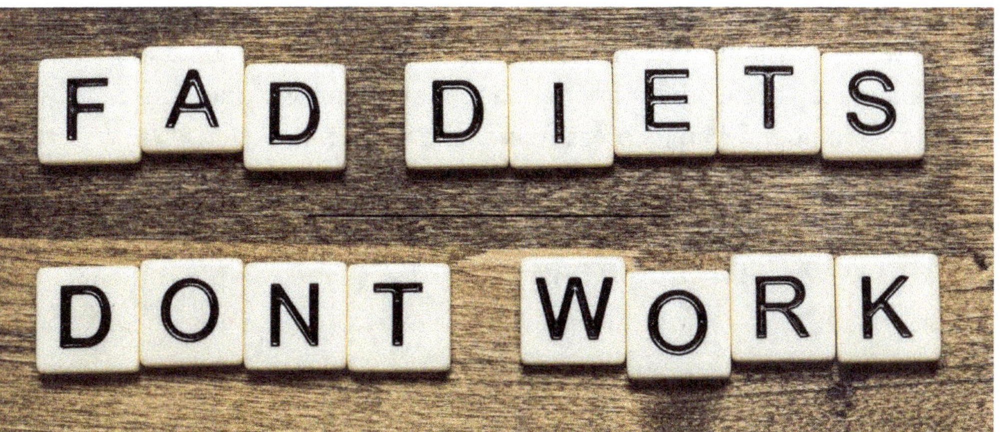


In today's world, it's not uncommon to hear about the latest trendy diet that promises quick and easy weight loss, improved health, and other health benefits.

Many of these diets claim to be backed by science or based on ancient wisdom, making them seem legitimate and trustworthy. It's no wonder that people are often drawn to these popular diet trends, hoping to achieve their desired results without too much effort.

However, while some popular diet trends may have some truth to them, many are not based on sound scientific evidence and can even be harmful to your health. It's important to understand the motivations behind why people are often drawn to these diets, as well as the potential risks and benefits of each diet trend.

Factors such as the desire for a quick fix, the fear of missing out (FOMO), and the influence of social media and celebrity endorsements can all contribute to the appeal of popular diet trends.

However, it's important to remember that what works for one person may not work for another, and that there is no one-size-fits-all solution when it comes to diet and nutrition.

## The Low-Carb Diet Trend

The low-carb diet trend has gained significant popularity in recent years, with many people following this approach for weight loss and overall health improvement.

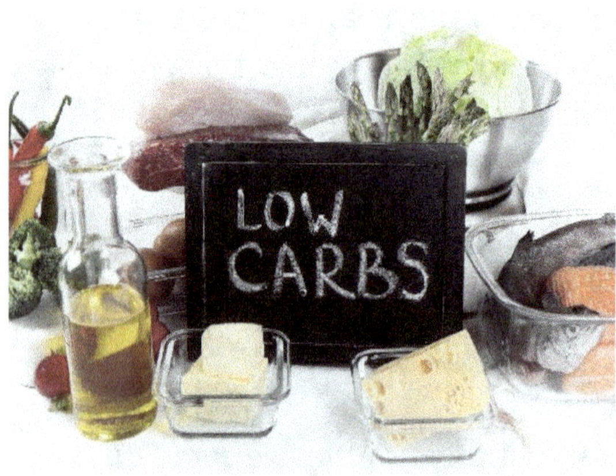


As the name suggests, the low-carb diet involves limiting the intake of carbohydrates and replacing them with protein and healthy fats.

The idea behind this diet is that reducing carbs will lower insulin levels, which in turn will force the body to burn stored fat for energy, resulting in weight loss.

The potential benefits of a low-carb diet are numerous. One of the most significant advantages is weight loss. By reducing the intake of carbohydrates, the body is forced to burn fat for energy, which can result in faster and more significant weight loss compared to other diets.

 Additionally, a low-carb diet can help lower blood sugar levels, reduce the risk of type 2 diabetes, and improve cholesterol levels.

However, there are also potential risks associated with a low-carb diet.

For instance, it may lead to nutritional deficiencies, particularly in fiber and essential vitamins and minerals found in fruits, whole grains, and starchy vegetables. Moreover, following a low-carb diet for a prolonged period may increase the risk of heart disease, kidney problems, and liver disease.

Despite the potential benefits and risks of the low-carb diet trend, many people choose to follow this approach due to its perceived effectiveness in weight loss and improved health. If you are considering a low-carb diet, it is essential to include healthy sources of protein and fats while limiting carbohydrates. Here are some examples of low-carb foods that you can include in your diet:

- **Eggs**: Eggs are an excellent source of protein and healthy fats, and they are low in carbs. You can enjoy boiled, scrambled, or as an omelet.

- **Nuts and seeds**: Nuts and seeds such as almonds, walnuts, and chia seeds are rich in healthy fats, protein, and fiber.

- **Leafy green vegetables**: Vegetables such as spinach, kale, and lettuce are low in carbs and rich in essential vitamins and minerals.

- **Lean meats**: Chicken, turkey, and beef are excellent sources of protein and healthy fats and are low in carbs.

- **Fish**: Fish such as salmon and tuna are rich in omega-3 fatty acids, which are beneficial for heart health and brain function. They are also low in carbs.

While the low-carb diet trend can offer some potential benefits for weight loss and improved health, it is essential to weigh the potential risks and consider a balanced approach to nutrition. Including healthy sources of protein, fats, and carbohydrates in your diet can help you achieve optimal health and wellness.

# The Plant-Based Diet Trend

The plant-based diet trend has gained popularity in recent years, with more people embracing the concept of a diet that focuses primarily on foods that come from plants, such as fruits, vegetables, whole grains, nuts, and seeds. This trend is often associated with a desire to improve health, reduce the risk of chronic diseases, and minimize one's impact on the environment.

One of the main potential benefits of a plant-based diet is that it tends to be high in fiber, vitamins, minerals, and antioxidants, all of which are essential for overall health and wellbeing. Research has shown that plant-based diets can reduce the risk of chronic diseases, such as heart disease, diabetes, and some types of cancer.

However, there are also potential risks associated with a plant-based diet, particularly if it is not well-planned. For example, some people may struggle to get enough protein or certain essential nutrients, such as vitamin B12, iron, and calcium, if they do not eat a variety of plant-based foods. It is essential to ensure that a plant-based diet includes a wide range of nutrient-dense foods to meet one's nutritional needs.

Some examples of plant-based foods and their health benefits include:

- **Leafy greens**: High in vitamins A, C, and K, as well as folate, fiber, and antioxidants. They can help reduce inflammation, support bone health, and improve digestion.

- **Berries**: Rich in antioxidants, fiber, and vitamin C. They may reduce the risk of heart disease, improve cognitive function, and help regulate blood sugar levels.

- **Legumes**: A good source of protein, fiber, iron, and other essential nutrients. They can help improve heart health, regulate blood sugar, and reduce the risk of certain cancers.

- **Whole grains**: Rich in fiber, vitamins, and minerals. They can help reduce the risk of heart disease, diabetes, and certain types of cancer.

- **Nuts and seeds**: High in healthy fats, protein, and fiber. They may improve heart health, regulate blood sugar, and support brain function.

The plant-based diet trend can have potential benefits for health and the environment, but it is essential to ensure that one's nutritional needs are met.

Eating a variety of plant-based foods can provide the body with essential nutrients and support overall health and wellbeing.

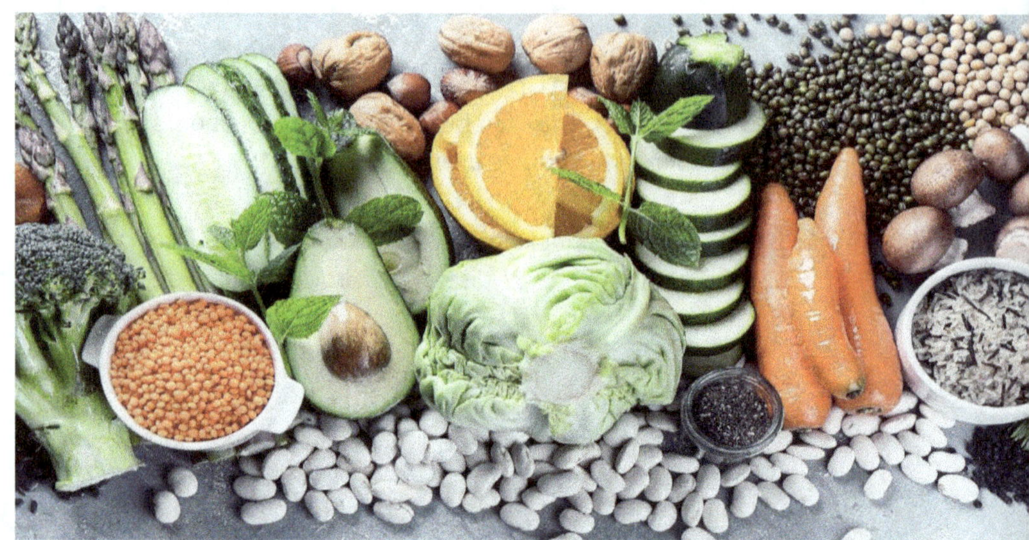

## The Intermittent Fasting Trend

Intermittent fasting is a diet trend that involves alternating periods of fasting and eating. There are various methods of intermittent fasting, but the most common ones are the 16/8 method, where one fasts for 16 hours and eats during an 8-hour window, and the 5:2 method, where one consumes a normal diet for 5 days and restricts calories to 500-600 for 2 days.

Proponents of intermittent fasting claim that it can help with weight loss, improve insulin sensitivity, reduce inflammation, and even increase lifespan. However, critics warn that it may lead to nutrient deficiencies, low energy levels, and binge-eating.

One of the main benefits of intermittent fasting is weight loss. By limiting the number of hours in which one can eat, the body is forced to burn stored fat for energy, resulting in weight loss.

It also improves insulin sensitivity, which can reduce the risk of type 2 diabetes.

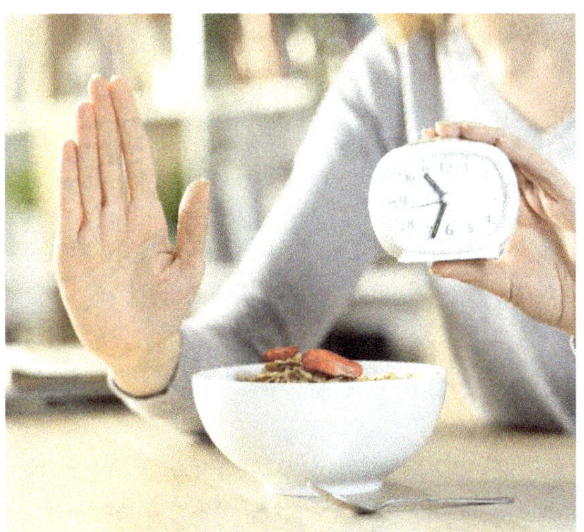

Additionally, intermittent fasting has been shown to reduce inflammation, which can help with various health conditions such as arthritis and heart disease.

However, there are also potential risks associated with intermittent fasting. For example, it may lead to nutrient deficiencies if one does not consume a balanced diet during the eating window.

It can also lead to low energy levels, which can affect one's ability to exercise and perform daily tasks. Furthermore, some people may be prone to binge-eating after a prolonged period of fasting, which can lead to weight gain.

During the eating window, it is important to consume nutrient-dense foods that can support health and well-being. Some examples of foods that can be consumed during intermittent fasting include lean proteins, whole grains, fruits, and vegetables. These foods can provide a variety of essential nutrients such as protein, fiber, vitamins, and minerals.

In conclusion, while intermittent fasting has been touted as a beneficial diet trend, it is important to weigh the potential benefits against the risks. It may be beneficial for some individuals, but not suitable for others.

It is important to consume nutrient-dense foods during the eating window and to consult with a healthcare professional before starting any new diet or exercise program.

## The Keto Diet Trend

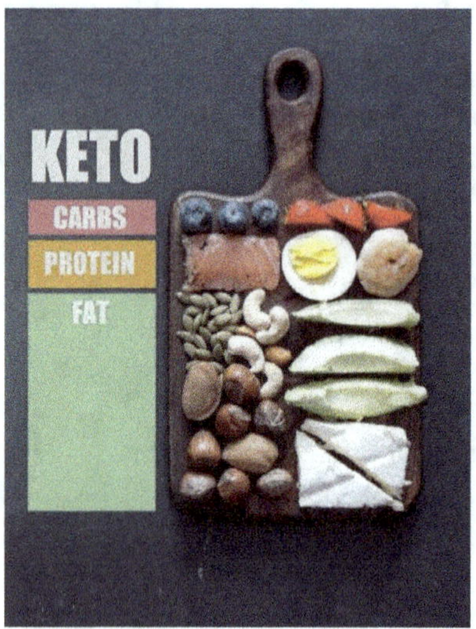


The ketogenic or keto diet is a popular diet trend that involves consuming high amounts of healthy fats, moderate protein, and very low carbohydrates. The primary goal of this diet is to achieve a state of ketosis, which is a metabolic state where the body burns fat for fuel instead of carbohydrates.

The keto diet has gained popularity in recent years for its potential benefits in weight loss, blood sugar control, and increased energy levels. However, like any diet trend, it has its potential risks and side effects.

One of the potential benefits of the keto diet is its ability to aid in weight loss. Since the body burns fat for fuel instead of carbohydrates, it can lead to significant weight loss. Additionally, the keto diet has shown potential in helping to regulate blood sugar levels, making it a viable option for those with type 2 diabetes.

Despite the potential benefits of the keto diet, there are also some risks associated with it. One of the primary concerns is that the diet is high in saturated fats, which can increase cholesterol levels and increase the risk of heart disease. Additionally, since the diet restricts carbohydrates, it can be challenging to get enough fiber and essential nutrients, leading to constipation and nutrient deficiencies.

To follow the keto diet, it's essential to consume foods that are high in healthy fats and low in carbohydrates. Some examples of keto-friendly foods include avocados, nuts and seeds, fatty fish, meat, cheese, and low-carb vegetables like spinach, broccoli, and cauliflower.

It's important to note that processed and sugary foods are not allowed on the keto diet, as they can lead to the body coming out of ketosis and negating the benefits of the diet.

In terms of health benefits, the keto diet has been shown to improve insulin sensitivity, reduce inflammation, and improve brain function. However, it's important to note that the diet is not suitable for everyone, especially those with liver or pancreatic issues. It's essential to speak with a healthcare provider before starting the keto diet to determine if it's safe and appropriate.

In conclusion, the keto diet is a popular diet trend that has shown potential benefits in weight loss, blood sugar control, and increased energy levels. However, it also has its potential risks and side effects, such as increased cholesterol levels and nutrient deficiencies.

To follow the keto diet, it's important to consume foods that are high in healthy fats and low in carbohydrates, while avoiding processed and sugary foods. It's essential to speak with a healthcare provider before starting the diet to determine if it's safe and appropriate.

# The Paleo Diet Trend

The paleo diet, also known as the caveman diet, is a popular diet trend that has gained popularity in recent years. The diet is based on the premise that our ancestors, who lived in the Paleolithic era, ate a diet that was primarily made up of meat, fish, fruits, and vegetables.

The paleo diet emphasizes eating whole, unprocessed foods and avoiding modern foods that were not available during the Paleolithic era, such as processed foods, grains, and dairy.

Advocates of the paleo diet argue that it can help people lose weight, improve their health, and reduce their risk of chronic diseases. However, the diet has also been criticized for being too restrictive and not providing enough essential nutrients.

Potential benefits of the paleo diet include weight loss, improved blood sugar control, and reduced inflammation. The diet is high in protein and fiber, which can help people feel full and reduce their overall calorie intake. It also eliminates processed foods and sugar, which are known to contribute to inflammation and chronic disease.

On the other hand, some experts warn that the paleo diet may be too restrictive and not provide enough essential nutrients.

Since the diet eliminates entire food groups like dairy and grains, it can be difficult for people to get enough calcium, vitamin D, and other important nutrients. Additionally, the diet can be high in saturated fat if people rely too heavily on meat for protein.

Some paleo-friendly foods include lean meats, fish, fruits, vegetables, nuts, and seeds. These foods are high in protein, fiber, and healthy fats, which can help people feel full and satisfied.

However, it's important to remember that the paleo diet should be customized to meet individual needs and preferences, and people should consult with a healthcare professional before making any significant dietary changes.

While the paleo diet has some potential health benefits, it's important to approach it with caution and to ensure that it provides a balanced and varied diet that meets all of the body's nutritional needs.

It's no secret that the world of nutrition and diet can be overwhelming and confusing. With new diets and trends popping up seemingly every day, it can be tempting to jump from one to the next in search of the "perfect" diet that promises quick and easy weight loss and optimal health.

However, it's important to remember that sustainable and balanced eating habits should be the foundation of any healthy diet, rather than relying on the latest trendy diet.

While trendy diets may promise quick and easy weight loss and other health benefits, they often come with risks and negative side effects. Instead, focusing on sustainable and balanced eating habits can lead to long-term health and wellness benefits, while also promoting a healthier relationship with food.

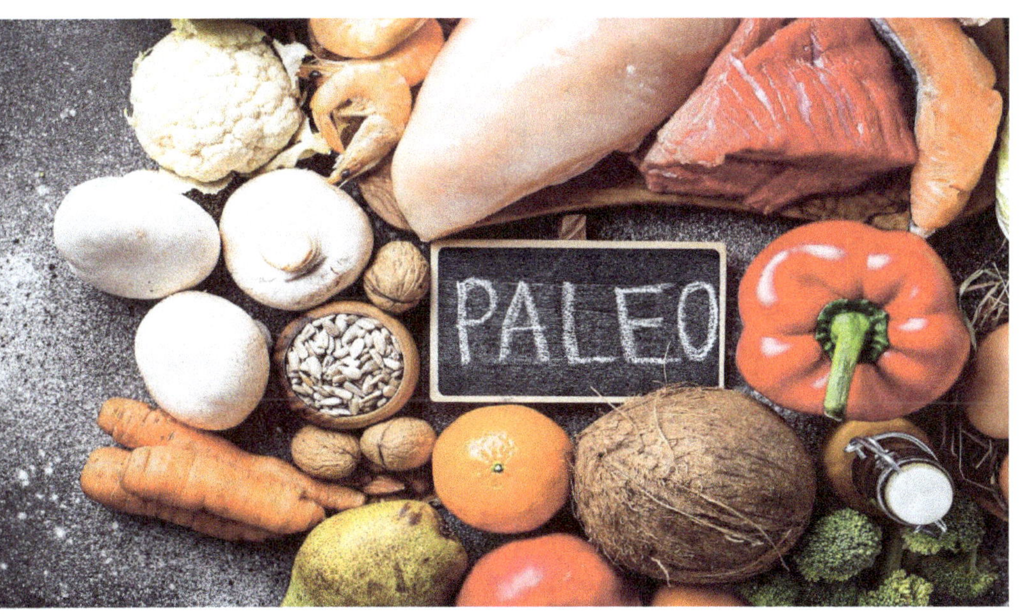

# Chapter 5: The Risks of Processed Foods

## What Are Processed Foods?

Processed foods refer to any food product that has been altered from its natural state through different methods such as canning, freezing, baking, and refining. In contrast, whole foods are those that are minimally processed or not processed at all and remain in their natural state.

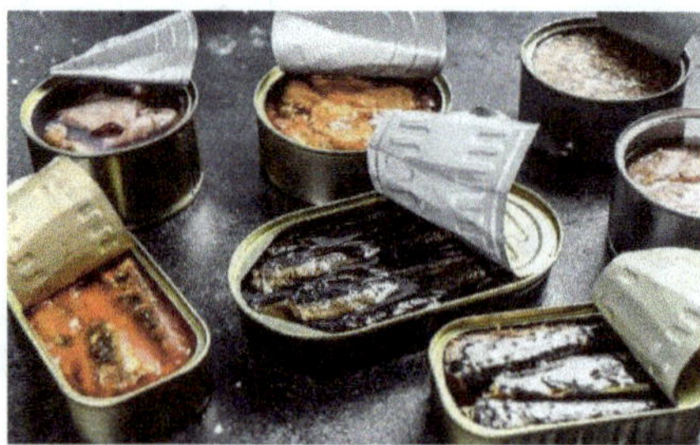

Processed foods are typically high in calories, unhealthy fats, sugar, salt, and additives, and low in essential nutrients such as vitamins, minerals, and fiber. They are often designed to be tasty, convenient, and have a longer shelf life, making them popular choices for people with busy lifestyles.

However, the process of refining and processing foods can strip them of their natural nutrients and fiber, leaving behind empty calories.

Whole foods, on the other hand, are packed with essential nutrients and fiber that are essential for optimal health. They include fruits, vegetables, whole grains, nuts, seeds, and legumes.

Whole foods are typically low in calories and fat, and high in fiber, vitamins, and minerals, making them ideal for maintaining a healthy weight and reducing the risk of chronic diseases.

In general, processed foods tend to be more convenient and affordable than whole foods, but they come with several downsides.

While whole foods nourish the body, processed foods may increase the risk of chronic diseases such as obesity, type 2 diabetes, heart disease, and some cancers. As such, it is crucial to understand the differences between processed and whole foods and prioritize consuming whole foods for optimal health.

## The Risks Associated with Processed Foods

Processed foods have become a staple in the modern diet due to their convenience, affordability, and availability. However, their consumption has been linked to negative health effects, particularly when consumed in excess. Processed foods are defined as food products that have undergone various processes, such as refining, preserving, and adding artificial ingredients, to increase their shelf life and improve their taste and texture. These processes can alter the nutritional content of the food, often reducing

g its fiber, vitamin, and mineral content while increasing its salt, sugar, and fat content.

The overconsumption of processed foods has been linked to numerous negative health effects, including weight gain, obesity, and related health issues. One reason for this is that processed foods are often high in calories, unhealthy fats, and added sugars, which can lead to increased calorie intake and contribute to weight gain. Additionally, these foods are often low in fiber and other essential nutrients, leading to nutrient deficiencies and poor overall health.

Processed foods have also been linked to an increased risk of chronic diseases such as type 2 diabetes, heart disease, and certain types of cancer.

This is because many processed foods contain high levels of artificial additives, such as preservatives, food dyes, and flavorings, which have been linked to these health issues. Moreover, the high salt content in processed foods has been linked to high blood pressure, which is a risk factor for heart disease.

One significant concern regarding processed foods is their potential to lead to overconsumption. Due to their high sugar, fat, and salt content, processed foods are often designed to be addictive, leading individuals to consume them in excess.

This can create a vicious cycle, with individuals consuming more and more processed foods to satisfy their cravings, which can contribute to weight gain and related health issues.

Processed foods are prevalent in the modern diet, and their consumption has been linked to negative health effects such as weight gain, obesity, and related health issues.

While it may be challenging to avoid processed foods entirely, individuals can take steps to reduce their consumption, such as choosing whole, unprocessed foods whenever possible, reading food labels carefully, and cooking meals at home using fresh, whole ingredients.

By making these changes, individuals can improve their overall health and reduce their risk of chronic diseases associated with processed food consumption.

# Tips for Reducing Processed Food Consumption

Ways to identify and avoid processed foods in the grocery store: One of the easiest ways to identify processed foods is to read the nutrition label. If the product contains a long list of artificial additives, preservatives, and added sugars, it is likely a processed food.

Another useful tip is to shop around the perimeter of the store, where the fresh produce, meat, and dairy products are located. Processed foods are often found in the center aisles, where they can be easily spotted due to their colorful packaging and marketing.

Tips for cooking and preparing whole foods at home: Cooking and preparing whole foods at home is a great way to reduce reliance on processed foods. Simple methods like roasting, steaming, and grilling can help retain the nutritional value of whole foods. It's also important to incorporate a variety of whole foods into your meals, including fruits, vegetables, whole grains, and lean proteins.

Experimenting with different herbs, spices, and sauces can help add flavor to your meals without relying on processed ingredients.

The importance of meal planning and preparation in reducing reliance on processed foods: Meal planning and preparation can help reduce reliance on processed foods by making it easier to cook and eat whole foods.

Planning meals ahead of time allows you to make a grocery list of whole foods, making it less likely that you'll buy processed foods on impulse. Meal prep can also help save time during the week by prepping ingredients or whole meals in advance.

**Ideas for healthy snacks and meals** that can be made with whole foods: There are many healthy snacks and meals that can be made with whole foods, such as:

- **Snacks**: sliced fruits and vegetables with hummus or nut butter, plain Greek yogurt with berries and nuts, whole grain crackers with avocado or guacamole.

- **Breakfast**: oatmeal with fruit and nuts, whole grain toast with avocado and eggs, smoothies with spinach, berries, and nut butter.

- **Lunch and dinner**: grilled chicken or fish with roasted vegetables, quinoa or brown rice bowls with mixed greens and avocado, vegetable stir-fry with brown rice, salads with a variety of vegetables and lean proteins.

Identifying and avoiding processed foods in the grocery store, cooking and preparing whole foods at home, meal planning and preparation, and incorporating healthy snacks and meals made with whole foods are all important steps in reducing reliance on processed foods.

By making these changes, individuals can improve their overall health and reduce the negative impact of processed foods on their well-being.

# Chapter 6: Food Additives: Understanding the Risks

Food additives are substances that are added to food products to improve their flavor, texture, color, or shelf life. There are many types of food additives, and they are often classified based on their function or origin.

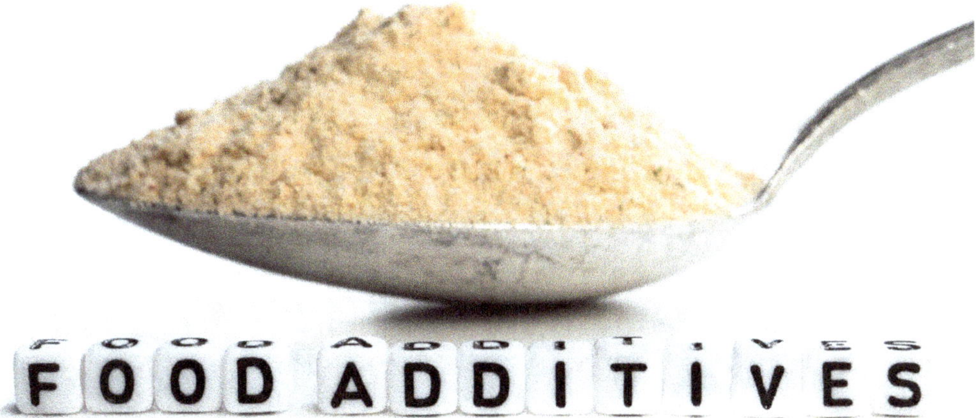



## Common Food Additives

Some common types of food additives include:

- **Preservatives**: These are additives that are added to foods to prevent spoilage and extend their shelf life. Examples include sodium benzoate, potassium sorbate, and sulfites.

- **Flavorings**: These are additives that are added to foods to enhance their taste or aroma. Examples include monosodium glutamate (MSG), artificial sweeteners, and natural flavors.

- **Colorants**: These are additives that are added to foods to improve their color or appearance. Examples include caramel color, titanium dioxide, and annatto.

- **Emulsifiers**: These are additives that are added to foods to help ingredients mix together more easily. Examples include lecithin, carrageenan, and xanthan gum.

- **Stabilizers**: These are additives that are added to foods to help maintain their texture or prevent separation. Examples include pectin, gelatin, and starches.

- **Nutrients**: These are additives that are added to foods to provide essential nutrients that may be lacking in the diet. Examples include vitamins, minerals, and fiber.

It's important to note that not all food additives are harmful, and some are even necessary for food safety and preservation. However, some additives have been linked to negative health effects, especially when consumed in large amounts over time.

Examples of common food additives that have raised concerns include high-fructose corn syrup, artificial colors and flavors, sodium nitrite, and monosodium glutamate (MSG).

It's important to read food labels and be aware of the types of additives in the foods you consume, and to limit your intake of those that have been linked to negative health effects.

## Risks Associated with Food Additives

Food additives are chemicals that are added to food to enhance its flavor, color, texture, and shelf life. While many of these additives are considered safe by regulatory bodies, there are some risks associated with their consumption.

Some of the common risks associated with food additives include:

1. **Allergic reactions**: Certain food additives can cause allergic reactions in some people. For example, sulfites, which are commonly used as preservatives, can cause an allergic reaction in people with asthma.

2. **Increased risk of cancer**: Some food additives, such as nitrates and nitrites, have been linked to an increased risk of cancer. These additives are commonly found in processed meats, such as hot dogs and bacon.

3. **Hormonal disruption**: Some food additives, such as bisphenol A (BPA) and phthalates, can disrupt hormone function in the body. BPA is commonly found in plastic food containers and can linings, while phthalates are found in plastic food packaging.

4. **Neurological effects**: Some food additives, such as monosodium glutamate (MSG), have been linked to neurological effects, including headaches and migraines.

5.  **Digestive issues**: Some food additives, such as artificial sweeteners, can cause digestive issues in some people. For example, some people may experience bloating or diarrhea after consuming products that contain certain artificial sweeteners.

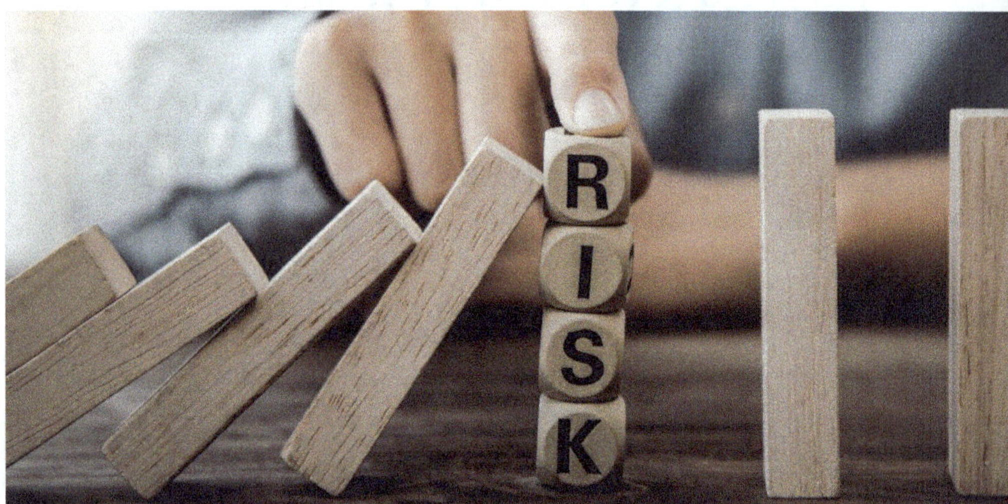


Overall, while many food additives are considered safe, it's important to be aware of the potential risks associated with their consumption.

To minimize the risks associated with food additives, it's important to read food labels carefully and avoid products that contain additives that you are sensitive to or that have been linked to health issues. Additionally, choosing whole, unprocessed foods whenever possible can help reduce your exposure to food additives.

# Regulations and Labeling Requirements

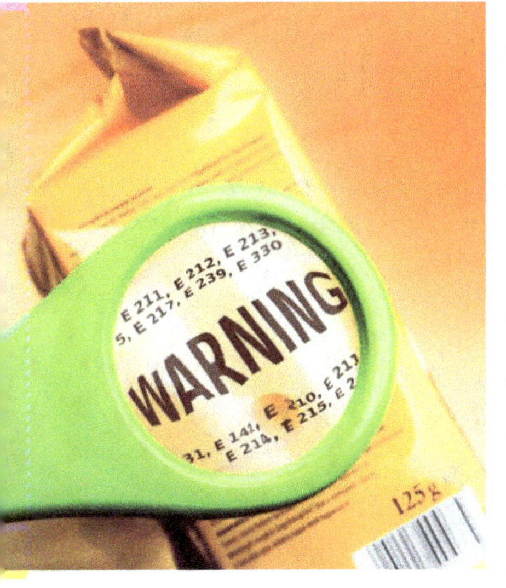


Regulations and labeling requirements are in place to ensure that food additives used in processed foods are safe for consumption and do not pose any health risks.

The U.S. Food and Drug Administration (FDA) is responsible for regulating food additives and ensuring their safety before they can be used in food products.

The FDA requires that all food additives undergo thorough testing and evaluation before they are approved for use in food products.

This testing includes determining the potential health effects of the additive, such as carcinogenicity, toxicity, and allergenicity.

Food manufacturers are required to list all ingredients on food labels, including any food additives used in the product. This allows consumers to make informed choices about the foods they purchase and consume.

In addition to listing the ingredients, food labels also provide information about the nutrient content of the food product. This information can be used to help consumers make healthier choices about the foods they eat.

It is important for consumers to read food labels carefully and to be aware of the various names that food additives may be listed under. For example, monosodium glutamate (MSG) may be listed as a flavor enhancer, while aspartame may be listed as a low-calorie sweetener.

Consumers can also look for labels on food products that indicate that the food is free of certain additives, such as artificial colors or flavors. Choosing foods that are free of certain additives can help reduce the risk of negative health effects associated with these additives.

Overall, regulations and labeling requirements are important tools for ensuring the safety of food additives and providing consumers with the information they need to make informed choices about the foods they consume.

## Ways to Avoid or Reduce Consumption of Food Additives

There are several ways to reduce consumption of food additives in our diet. Here are some tips:

- **Choose whole, unprocessed foods**: By choosing fresh fruits, vegetables, whole grains, and unprocessed meats, you can avoid many of the food additives found in processed foods.

- **Read food labels**: Be aware of the ingredients listed on food labels, and choose products with minimal or no additives. Avoid foods with long ingredient lists or those with additives you don't recognize or can't pronounce.

- **Buy organic**: Organic foods are grown without the use of synthetic pesticides, fertilizers, or other harmful chemicals that may contain additives. However, organic foods can still contain some additives, so it is important to read labels.

- **Cook meals at home**: Preparing your meals from scratch allows you to control the ingredients and avoid unnecessary additives.

Try using fresh herbs and spices for flavor instead of processed seasoning blends.



- **Limit processed and packaged foods**: Processed and packaged foods are often high in additives. Try to limit your consumption of these types of foods and choose fresh, whole foods instead.

- **Choose natural alternatives**: When cooking or baking, try using natural alternatives to food additives. For example, use honey or maple syrup instead of artificial sweeteners, or use apple cider vinegar as a natural preservative.

- **Be aware of hidden sources of additives**: Additives can also be found in products such as vitamins, medications, and supplements. Be sure to read labels and research products before consuming them.

By following these tips, you can reduce your consumption of food additives and make healthier food choices.

# Chapter 7: Practical Meal Planning Tips for Healthy Eating

Meal planning is an essential tool for maintaining a healthy and balanced diet while saving time and money. It involves the process of planning and preparing meals ahead of time, often for a week or more.

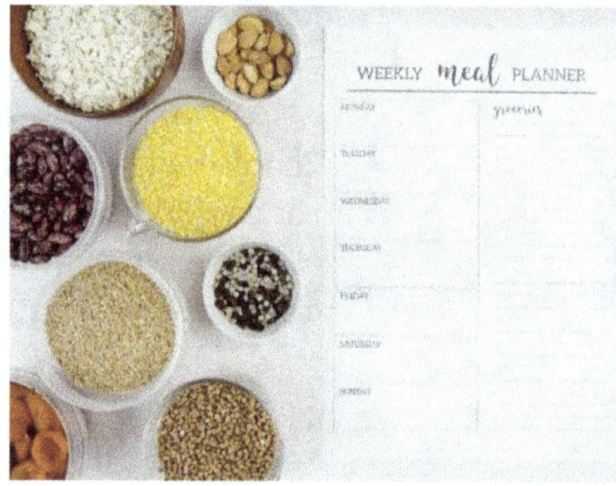

Meal planning can help individuals make healthier food choices, reduce food waste, and save money by avoiding unnecessary purchases.

Additionally, planning meals can also help individuals to stay on track with their dietary goals and prevent impulse eating.

## Setting Meal Planning Goals

Setting meal planning goals can be an effective way to achieve healthy eating habits. Before starting meal planning, it's important to identify specific goals and the reasons behind them. This can help provide motivation and make the process more meaningful.

Goals can vary based on individual needs and preferences. For some, the goal may be to increase the intake of vegetables or to reduce the consumption of processed foods. Others may focus on meal prepping or reducing food waste. It's important to keep in mind that goals should be realistic and achievable.

Once goals have been established, they can be used as a guide when selecting recipes and planning meals. For example, if the goal is to increase vegetable intake, a meal plan may include more salads or vegetable-based soups. If the goal is to reduce processed foods, meals can be centered around whole foods such as fruits, vegetables, and lean proteins.

By keeping goals in mind during meal planning, it can be easier to make healthier choices and stick to a nutritious diet. Additionally, setting goals can provide a sense of accomplishment and motivation to continue with healthy habits.

## Strategies for Meal Planning

One strategy for meal planning is to **create a weekly meal plan**. This involves deciding on the meals you will eat for the entire week and creating a shopping list for the necessary ingredients. This strategy can help you avoid the temptation of eating unhealthy foods, reduce food waste, and save money by buying ingredients in bulk.

Another strategy is to **meal prep**. This involves preparing meals in advance and storing them in the fridge or freezer to be reheated later. Meal prepping can save you time during busy weekdays and ensure that you have healthy meals readily available when you need them.

**Batch cooking** is another meal planning strategy. This involves preparing large batches of food and dividing them into portions for future meals. Batch cooking can be especially useful for foods that can be frozen, such as soups, stews, and casseroles.

Finally, incorporating theme nights into your meal plan can help add variety and fun to your meal planning. For example, you could have a Mexican-themed night, Italian-themed night, or vegetarian-themed night. This strategy can also help simplify meal planning by grouping similar meals together.

## Tips for Healthy Meal Preparation

Preparing healthy meals is an essential part of achieving a balanced and nutritious diet. However, it can be challenging to prepare healthy meals consistently, especially when life gets busy. Here are some tips for healthy meal preparation:

1. **Plan ahead**: Planning ahead can help ensure that you have all the necessary ingredients and equipment for meal preparation. Consider setting aside a few hours each week for meal planning and preparation.

2. **Choose healthy ingredients**: Choose ingredients that are fresh and nutrient-dense. Include a variety of fruits, vegetables, whole grains, lean proteins, and healthy fats in your meals.

3. **Use healthy cooking methods**: Choose cooking methods that preserve the nutrients in the food, such as steaming, grilling, or roasting. Avoid deep-frying or using excessive amounts of oil.

4. **Practice portion control**: Use measuring cups and spoons to ensure that you are eating the appropriate portion sizes. It can be easy to overeat when portions are not controlled.

5.  **Pack meals ahead of time**: Preparing meals in advance can save time and ensure that you have healthy meals ready to eat during busy days. Use meal prep containers to pack and store your meals in the fridge or freezer.

6.  **Experiment with healthy recipes**: Trying new recipes can help keep meal preparation interesting and enjoyable. Look for recipes that include healthy ingredients and are easy to prepare.

By incorporating these tips into your daily routine, you can make healthy eating a sustainable habit for the long-term.

Remember, small changes can add up over time and lead to significant improvements in your health and well-being.

So, don't be afraid to experiment, try new things, and enjoy the journey towards a healthier you.

# Chapter 8: Superfoods: The Health Benefits of Eating Fruits

Fruits are not only nature's sweet and refreshing treats, but they also possess an incredible array of health benefits. Packed with vitamins, minerals, fiber, and antioxidants, fruits offer a unique combination of nutrients that can contribute to overall well-being.

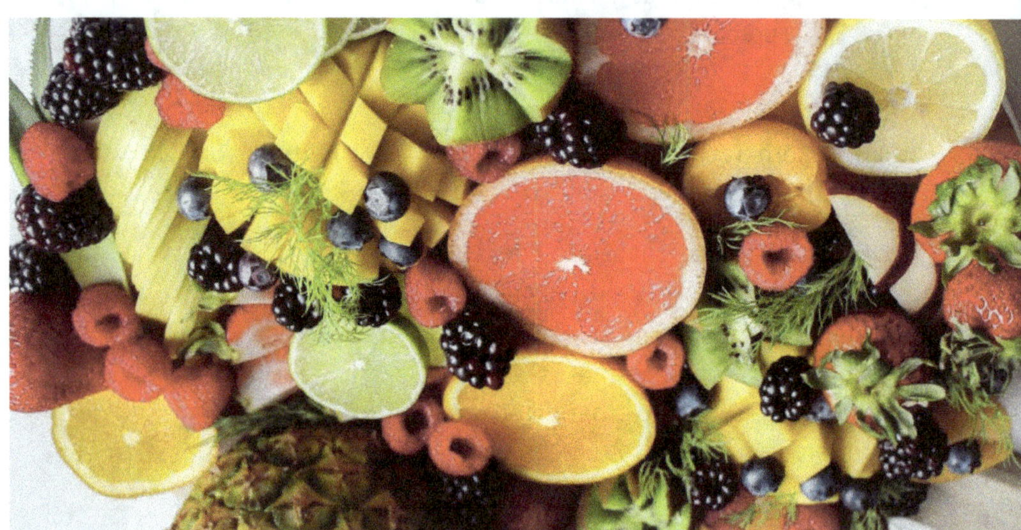

 Incorporating a variety of fruits into your daily diet can have a profound impact on your health and vitality.

One of the remarkable aspects of fruits is their rich content of essential vitamins and minerals. These nutrients play a crucial role in supporting various bodily functions and maintaining optimal health. From vitamin C in citrus fruits that boosts immune function to potassium in bananas that supports heart health, each fruit brings its own set of nutrients to the table.

In addition to vitamins and minerals, fruits are abundant in dietary fiber. Fiber aids in digestion, helps regulate blood sugar levels, and promotes feelings of fullness, making it beneficial for weight management.

Furthermore, the natural sugars found in fruits are accompanied by fiber, which slows down their absorption, preventing rapid spikes in blood sugar levels.

Another exceptional feature of fruits is their high antioxidant content. Antioxidants help protect the body against harmful free radicals, which can cause oxidative stress and contribute to chronic diseases. By consuming a variety of colorful fruits, you can ensure a diverse range of antioxidants that provide powerful defense against cellular damage.

Moreover, fruits are hydrating due to their high-water content, which supports overall hydration and contributes to healthy skin and a refreshed complexion.

The combination of water, fiber, and natural sugars in fruits also makes them a fantastic choice for replenishing energy levels and staying hydrated throughout the day.

To reap the full benefits of fruits, it's essential to include a diverse selection in your diet. Each fruit brings its own unique set of health-promoting compounds and flavors, so try to incorporate a rainbow of colors on your plate.

From berries bursting with antioxidants to tropical fruits abundant in vitamin C, embracing variety is key.

By embracing the power of fruits and incorporating them into your daily diet, you can enhance your overall health and well-being. Enjoy them as a refreshing snack, blend them into smoothies, or use them to add natural sweetness to your favorite recipes. The possibilities are endless, and the benefits are immense.

Remember, when it comes to fruits, diversity is key.

Explore the vibrant world of fruits, savor their flavors, and relish in the incredible health benefits they have to offer. Your body will thank you for nourishing it with the power of fruits.

## Nutrient-Rich Superfruits: Blueberries, Strawberries, and Pomegranates

Superfruits are a category of fruits that go above and beyond when it comes to their nutritional value and health benefits. Among these superfruits, blueberries, strawberries, and pomegranates stand out as nutritional powerhouses, offering a wealth of nutrients that can greatly contribute to your well-being.

Let's start with **blueberries**, often referred to as "nature's candy." These small berries are packed with antioxidants that help combat oxidative stress and protect against cellular damage. Blueberries are also rich in vitamin C, which supports immune function, and dietary fiber, which aids in digestion and promotes a healthy gut. Additionally, their deep blue color is attributed to anthocyanins, compounds that have been linked to improved brain function and memory.

**Strawberries**, with their vibrant red hue and sweet flavor, are not only delicious but also highly nutritious. They are an excellent source of vitamin C, known for its immune-boosting properties and role in collagen production. Strawberries also contain folate, which plays a crucial role in cell division and DNA synthesis. Furthermore, their high antioxidant content helps reduce inflammation in the body and supports cardiovascular health.

**Pomegranates**, with their unique ruby-red arils, have long been regarded as a symbol of health and fertility. These jewel-like seeds are rich in antioxidants, particularly punicalagins, which have been associated with reducing inflammation and protecting against heart disease. Pomegranates also contain polyphenols, which have been shown to have anticancer properties. Additionally, this superfruit is a good source of vitamins C and K, as well as fiber, making it a valuable addition to a nutritious diet.

Incorporating these nutrient-rich superfruits into your diet can have a significant impact on your overall health. Whether enjoyed on their own, added to smoothies, or used as toppings for yogurt or oatmeal, these superfruits offer a burst of flavor and a wealth of health-enhancing properties. Including them in your daily routine can provide a range of benefits, from boosting your immune system to supporting heart health and cognitive function.

## Remember that variety is key!

While blueberries, strawberries, and pomegranates are known for their exceptional nutritional profiles, there are many other superfruits worth exploring, such as acai berries, goji berries, and cranberries. Embrace the abundance of nature's superfruits and let their vibrant colors and delightful flavors nourish your body and invigorate your health.

# Exploring the Health Benefits of Fruits: Strengthening the Immune System, Protecting the Heart, and Promoting Digestive Health

Fruits are not only nature's sweet treats; they also offer a myriad of health benefits that can enhance our overall well-being.

First and foremost, fruits are packed with immune-boosting properties. Rich in essential vitamins, minerals, and antioxidants, they provide a wide range of nutrients that support immune function and help ward off infections and diseases. Vitamin C, found abundantly in citrus fruits like oranges and grapefruits, is a powerful antioxidant that aids in strengthening the immune system and fighting off harmful pathogens

. Additionally, fruits like berries, kiwis, and papayas are rich in antioxidants that combat oxidative stress, reduce inflammation, and support a healthy immune response.

When it comes to heart health, certain fruits have shown remarkable protective effects. Grapes, for example, contain a high concentration of antioxidants known as polyphenols, particularly resveratrol, which has been linked to cardiovascular benefits.

These antioxidants help reduce inflammation, lower blood pressure, and improve overall heart function. Similarly, citrus fruits like oranges and lemons are packed with vitamin C and flavonoids, which have been associated with a reduced risk of heart disease.

Regular consumption of these fruits can contribute to a healthy heart and a reduced likelihood of cardiovascular issues.

In addition to boosting the immune system and protecting the heart, fruits play a crucial role in promoting digestive health. Many fruits are rich in dietary fiber, which aids in proper digestion, prevents constipation, and supports a healthy gut.

Fiber acts as a prebiotic, nourishing the beneficial bacteria in our intestines and promoting a balanced gut microbiome. Fruits such as apples, bananas, and berries are excellent sources of fiber and can help regulate bowel movements and improve overall gut function.

Incorporating a variety of fruits into your diet is a wonderful way to harness their health-promoting benefits. Whether enjoyed as a refreshing snack, blended into smoothies, or added to salads and desserts, fruits offer a natural and delicious way to strengthen the immune system, protect the heart, and promote digestive health.

Experiment with different types of fruits to enjoy a wide range of nutrients and flavors, and aim to include them in your daily meals and snacks.

By embracing the power of fruits, you can nourish your body with an abundance of vitamins, minerals, antioxidants, and fiber. These nutritional powerhouses support your immune system, protect your heart, and promote optimal digestive health.

Explore the vibrant world of fruits and unlock their potential to enhance your overall well-being. Your body will thank you for the colorful and delicious gift of nature's bounty.

# Incorporating Superfruits into Your Diet: Practical tips and creative ideas for incorporating a variety of superfruits into your daily meals and snacks.

One simple way to enjoy superfruits is by adding them to your **morning routine**. Kickstart your day with a nutrient-packed breakfast by topping your cereal or oatmeal with a handful of fresh blueberries or strawberries. You can also blend these superfruits into smoothies for a refreshing and energizing start to your day. Consider combining them with other fruits, yogurt, and a dash of honey for a delightful burst of flavors.

For a **midday pick-me-up**, create fruit-infused water by adding slices of citrus fruits, such as oranges or lemons, to a pitcher of water. Not only does this add a refreshing twist to your hydration routine, but it also infuses the water with the invigorating flavors and immune-boosting properties of these superfruits. Keep a bottle of this revitalizing beverage with you throughout the day to stay hydrated and nourished.

Superfruits can also be incorporated into your **lunch and dinner** recipes to elevate both the taste and nutritional value of your meals. Add a handful of pomegranate arils to a colorful salad for a delightful burst of sweetness and a dose of antioxidants. Sprinkle fresh berries over a bed of mixed greens, or blend them into a homemade vinaigrette for a tangy twist.

You can also include sliced strawberries or blueberries in your savory dishes, such as grilled chicken or roasted vegetables, to add a hint of natural sweetness and a vibrant touch.

**Snack time** is another opportunity to enjoy the benefits of superfruits. Keep a stash of dried berries or freeze-dried fruits in your pantry for a quick and nutritious snack on the go. You can also create your own fruit parfait by layering Greek yogurt, granola, and a medley of sliced superfruits. The combination of creamy yogurt and vibrant fruits provides a satisfying and nourishing snack that will keep you energized throughout the day.

Remember to explore the seasonal availability of superfruits and incorporate them into your meals accordingly. Whether enjoyed fresh, frozen, or dried, superfruits can be a versatile addition to your culinary repertoire.

Get creative with your recipes, experiment with different combinations, and savor the vibrant flavors and health benefits they offer.

# Chapter 9: Superfoods: The Health Benefits of Eating Vegetables

Incorporating vegetables into a healthy diet is a fundamental step towards achieving optimal health and well-being. Vegetables are nature's powerhouses, packed with essential nutrients, vitamins, minerals, and antioxidants that promote overall vitality and support the proper functioning of the body.

These vibrant and colorful gems of nature offer a multitude of health benefits and play a crucial role in disease prevention, weight management, and maintaining a strong immune system.

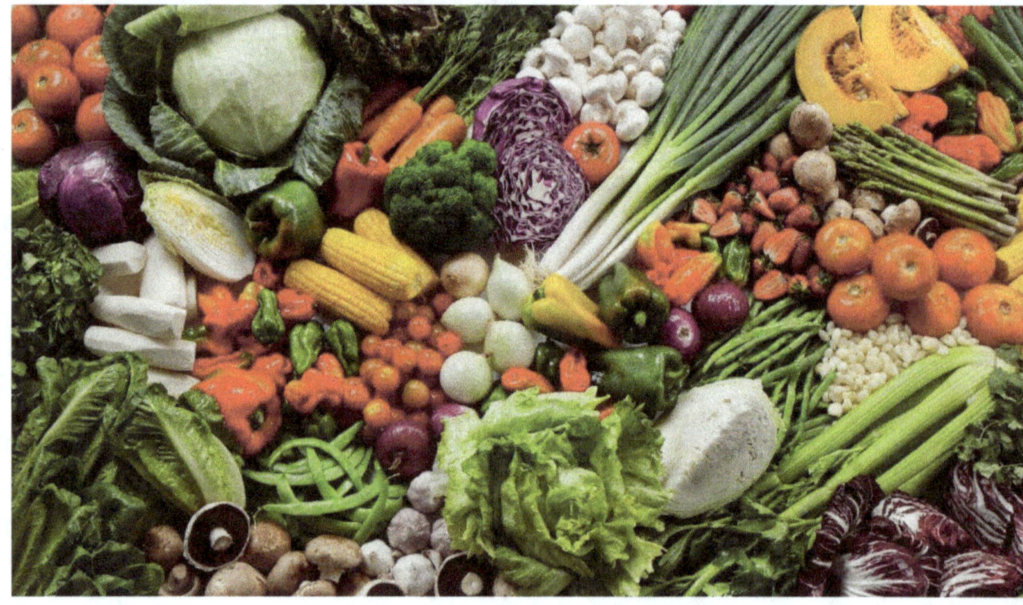

Vegetables are an incredible source of fiber, which aids in digestion, promotes satiety, and helps maintain a healthy weight. They are also rich in vitamins, such as vitamin C, vitamin A, and vitamin K, which support immune function, vision, and bone health, respectively.

Additionally, vegetables provide an abundance of minerals like potassium, magnesium, and folate, which are essential for cardiovascular health, energy production, and cell growth.

## Nutrient-Rich Powerhouses

Vegetables are nutrient-rich powerhouses that offer a wide array of essential vitamins, minerals, and antioxidants. Leafy greens like spinach and kale are packed with vitamin K, which supports bone health and blood clotting.

Orange and yellow vegetables, such as carrots and sweet potatoes, are rich in beta-carotene, a precursor to vitamin A that promotes healthy vision and skin.

Cruciferous vegetables like broccoli and cauliflower contain sulforaphane, a compound with potent anti-cancer properties. These are just a few examples of the diverse nutrients found in vegetables that contribute to overall health and well-being.

## Prevention and Management of Chronic Diseases:

Research consistently demonstrates that incorporating a variety of vegetables into your diet can help prevent and manage chronic diseases. The rich antioxidant content of vegetables helps combat oxidative stress, a major contributor to heart disease, diabetes, and certain types of cancer.

The fiber content in vegetables supports healthy digestion, reduces the risk of colorectal cancer, and helps control blood sugar levels.

Additionally, the phytochemicals present in vegetables have been linked to a lower risk of chronic diseases, including cardiovascular disease and neurodegenerative disorders.

## Weight Management and Satiety:

Vegetables play a crucial role in weight management and promoting satiety. They are low in calories and high in fiber, which helps control appetite and keeps you feeling fuller for longer.

By including vegetables in your meals, you can increase the volume of your plate without significantly increasing the calorie content.

The high fiber content of vegetables also aids in maintaining a healthy weight by regulating blood sugar levels and preventing overeating.

Adding a variety of colorful vegetables to your meals ensures a nutrient-dense and satisfying eating experience while supporting weight management goals.

## Exploring Superstar (Superfood) Vegetables:

When it comes to superfoods, certain vegetables stand out as nutritional powerhouses, offering an abundance of health benefits.

Let's take a closer look at some superstar vegetables that have gained recognition for their unique nutritional profile and potential health-enhancing properties.

- **Kale**: This leafy green vegetable has gained tremendous popularity for its exceptional nutrient density. It is packed with vitamins A, C, and K, along with minerals like calcium and potassium. Kale is known for its anti-inflammatory properties, thanks to its high antioxidant content. It supports eye health, strengthens the immune system, and promotes cardiovascular health.

- **Spinach**: Another green leafy vegetable that deserves the spotlight is spinach. It is an excellent source of vitamins A, C, and K, as well as folate and iron. Spinach is known for its role in promoting bone health, supporting brain function, and providing a good dose of antioxidants that help combat oxidative stress and inflammation.

- **Broccoli**: This cruciferous vegetable is rich in fiber, vitamins C and K, and various antioxidants. Broccoli contains a compound called sulforaphane, which has been studied for its anti-cancer properties. It supports detoxification processes in the body, promotes heart health, and provides immune-boosting benefits.

- **Sweet Potatoes**: These vibrant root vegetables are not only delicious but also highly nutritious. They are a great source of vitamins A and C, potassium, and fiber. Sweet potatoes are known for their antioxidant content and their ability to support eye health, boost the immune system, and contribute to healthy digestion.

Each of these superstar vegetables offers a unique nutritional profile and a range of potential health benefits. By incorporating them into your diet, you can elevate your nutrient intake and enjoy their remarkable properties.

So, let these superstar vegetables take center stage in your meals, adding both flavor and exceptional health benefits to your plate.

# Creative Ways to Incorporate Vegetables

Incorporating vegetables into your meals and snacks doesn't have to be a monotonous or boring task. With a little creativity, you can elevate the taste, texture, and visual appeal of your dishes while enjoying the numerous health benefits of vegetables.

Here are some practical tips and creative ideas to help you incorporate more vegetables into your daily routine:

1. **Veggie-packed smoothies**: Add a handful of leafy greens like spinach or kale to your fruit smoothies. The mild taste of fruits will mask the flavor of the vegetables while providing an extra dose of vitamins and minerals.

2. **Spiralized vegetables**: Invest in a spiralizer to transform vegetables like zucchini, carrots, or sweet potatoes into noodle-like strands. Use them as a base for stir-fries, salads, or even as a substitute for pasta.

3. **Veggie-loaded omelets and frittatas**: Whip up a nutritious breakfast by adding sautéed vegetables such as bell peppers, mushrooms, spinach, or onions to your omelets or frittatas. It's a delicious way to start your day with a boost of vitamins and fiber.

4. **Veggie dips and spreads**: Blend roasted or steamed vegetables like cauliflower, eggplant, or carrots with herbs, spices, and a

touch of olive oil to create flavorful and nutritious dips or spreads. Enjoy them with whole-grain crackers or raw veggie sticks.

5. **Sneak vegetables into sauces and soups**: Puree cooked vegetables like carrots, butternut squash, or cauliflower and incorporate them into sauces, soups, or stews. It adds richness, creaminess, and an extra nutritional punch to your dishes.

6. **Vegetable wraps and lettuce cups**: Swap out tortillas or bread with large lettuce leaves or collard greens to create delicious and refreshing wraps. Fill them with a variety of colorful vegetables, lean protein, and your favorite sauces or dressings.

7. **Grilled or roasted vegetable skewers**: Thread an assortment of vegetables onto skewers, brush them with a little olive oil, and grill or roast them for a flavorful and nutritious side dish. It's a great way to add a burst of color and variety to your meals.

8. **Veggie-centric salads:** Build vibrant salads by combining a variety of vegetables, leafy greens, nuts, seeds, and a tangy vinaigrette. Experiment with different textures, flavors, and colors to create visually appealing and satisfying salads.

Remember, the key to incorporating more vegetables into your meals is to experiment, have fun, and embrace the versatility of vegetables.

By getting creative with your cooking techniques and recipes, you'll discover new ways to enjoy the goodness of vegetables while nourishing your body with essential nutrients.

Incorporating vegetables into your diet is a powerful step towards achieving a nourishing and vibrant lifestyle.

By exploring the wide array of vegetables available and experimenting with different recipes and cooking techniques, you could discover your favorite flavors and unleash your culinary creativity.

Vegetables provide a rich source of essential nutrients, fiber, and antioxidants that support overall health and well-being.

They play a crucial role in preventing and managing chronic diseases, supporting weight management, and promoting satiety.

From nutrient-rich powerhouses to superstar vegetables like kale, spinach, broccoli, and sweet potatoes, each vegetable brings its unique nutritional profile and potential health-enhancing properties to the table.

By embracing vegetables as the foundation of your meals, you not only add vibrancy and variety to your plate but also empower yourself to make informed choices that benefit your overall health. Get creative with veggie-packed smoothies, spiralized vegetables, and veggie-loaded omelets.

Explore the world of vegetable dips, sauces, and soups. Enjoy the crunch of vegetable wraps, the sizzle of grilled skewers, and the freshness of veggie-centric salads.

In this journey towards a healthier lifestyle, remember to experiment, have fun, and let your taste buds guide you. Each vegetable offers a unique flavor, texture, and nutritional profile, so don't be afraid to try new varieties and combinations.

Empower yourself with the knowledge that vegetables have the power to nourish and revitalize your body.

So, let your imagination run wild in the kitchen and embrace the incredible diversity of vegetables. Discover your favorites, create delicious meals, and experience the transformative impact of incorporating more vegetables into your daily life.

Let vegetables be the hero of your plate and the key to unlocking a nourishing and vibrant diet. Your body and taste buds will thank you!

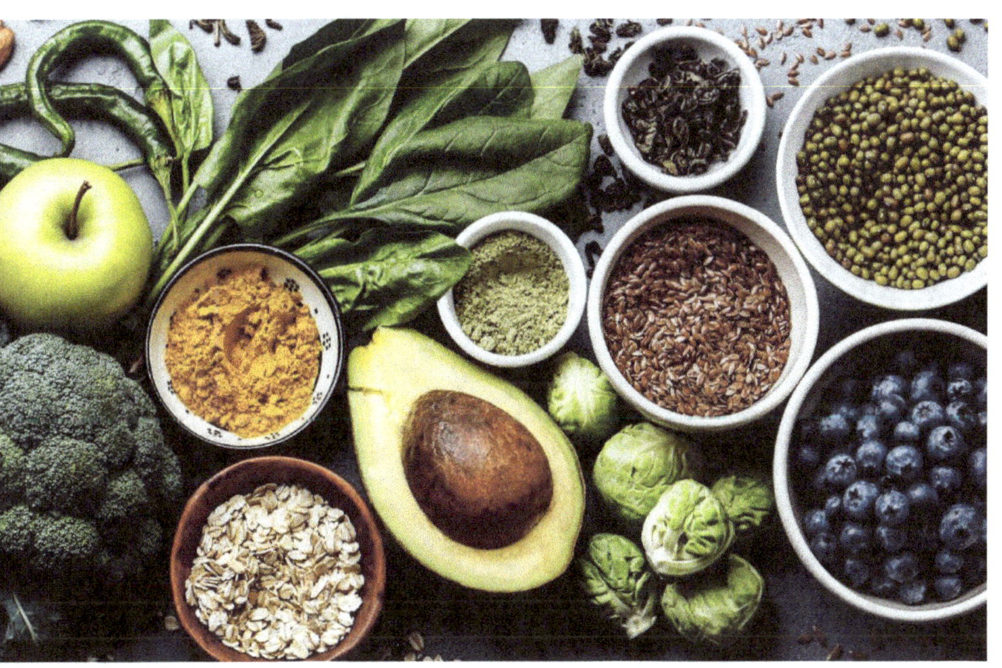

# Chapter 10: The Best Protein Sources for Healthy Living

Protein is an essential nutrient that plays a vital role in supporting overall health and well-being. It serves as the building block for our cells, tissues, and organs, and is involved in various critical functions in the body.

From repairing and building muscles to supporting immune function and regulating hormones, protein is a key player in maintaining optimal health.

One of the primary functions of protein is its role in tissue repair and growth. It is responsible for repairing damaged tissues, building new cells, and supporting the growth and maintenance of muscles, bones, and skin. Protein also plays a crucial role in the production of enzymes, hormones, and antibodies that are essential for various metabolic processes and immune function.

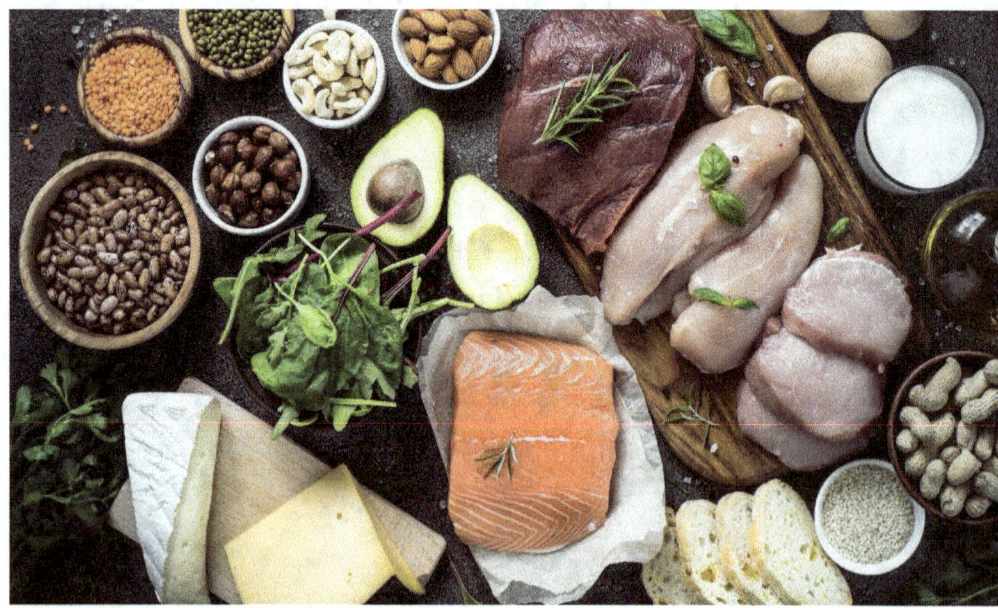

Protein is a macronutrient that provides the body with energy. Unlike carbohydrates and fats, protein is not the body's primary source of energy, but it serves as a backup fuel source when carbohydrates are limited.

This makes protein an important nutrient for maintaining energy levels and supporting physical endurance.

Additionally, protein plays a significant role in weight management. It is known to promote feelings of fullness and satiety, which can help control appetite and prevent overeating.

Including adequate protein in your meals and snacks can help regulate blood sugar levels, curb cravings, and support weight loss or maintenance goals.

Protein is found in both animal and plant-based sources, and it's important to consume a variety of protein-rich foods to ensure a balanced and complete amino acid profile. Lean meats, poultry, fish, dairy products, legumes, nuts, and seeds are all excellent sources of protein.

## Animal-Based Protein Sources:

Animal-based protein sources are derived from animal products and are considered complete proteins as they contain all the essential amino acids required by the body. Lean meats such as poultry, beef, pork, and lamb are excellent sources of high-quality protein.

They provide essential nutrients like iron, vitamin B12, and zinc. Fish and seafood are also rich in protein and contain beneficial omega-3 fatty acids, which are important for heart health.

Dairy products such as milk, yogurt, and cheese are another source of animal-based protein. They provide calcium, vitamin D, and other essential nutrients along with protein. Eggs are a versatile and nutrient-dense source of protein, containing all the essential amino acids.

# Plant-Based Protein Sources:

Plant-based protein sources are derived from plant foods and can provide adequate protein when combined strategically. Legumes, including beans, lentils, chickpeas, and peas, are excellent sources of plant-based protein.

They are also rich in fiber, vitamins, and minerals. Nuts and seeds, such as almonds, walnuts, chia seeds, and flaxseeds, contain protein and healthy fats. Additionally, they offer other beneficial nutrients like omega-3 fatty acids and antioxidants.

Whole grains like quinoa, brown rice, and oats also contribute to the daily protein intake. They provide a decent amount of protein and are high in fiber and other essential nutrients.

Certain vegetables like spinach, broccoli, and Brussels sprouts also contain protein in smaller amounts, along with various vitamins, minerals, and antioxidants.

# Combining Protein Sources for Complete Nutrition:

Combining different protein sources can ensure that you obtain a wide range of amino acids and achieve a complete and balanced protein intake.

For individuals following a vegetarian or vegan diet, it is especially important to combine plant-based protein sources to obtain all the essential amino acids.

One strategy is to combine legumes with grains, such as beans with rice or lentils with quinoa. This combination creates a complete protein profile, providing all the essential amino acids your body needs.

Additionally, including a variety of plant-based protein sources throughout the day, such as legumes, nuts, seeds, and whole grains, can help ensure you receive a diverse array of nutrients along with your protein intake.

## Meeting Protein Needs for Different Lifestyles:

Protein needs vary depending on factors such as age, gender, activity level, and overall health. It is important to assess your individual protein requirements and adjust your intake accordingly.

For sedentary individuals, the recommended daily protein intake is around 0.8 grams of protein per kilogram of body weight.

However, for those who are physically active, such as athletes or individuals engaged in strength training, protein needs may be higher to support muscle repair and growth. In such cases, protein intake may range from 1.2 to 2.0 grams of protein per kilogram of body weight.

It is also important to consider protein needs during specific life stages, such as pregnancy or older adulthood, where protein requirements may be increased for proper growth, development, and maintenance of muscle mass.

By understanding your specific protein needs and incorporating a variety of protein sources into your diet, you can ensure that you are meeting your nutritional requirements for optimal health and well-being.

# Plant-Based Protein for Vegetarians and Vegans:

Vegetarians and vegans have a plethora of options to meet their protein needs through plant-based sources. A diverse range of plant-based protein sources can provide all the essential amino acids required for optimal health.

Legumes, including beans, lentils, and chickpeas, are not only rich in protein but also offer a significant amount of fiber, vitamins, and minerals.

Tofu, tempeh, and seitan are popular plant-based protein choices that provide a meat-like texture and can be used in various recipes, from stir-fries to burgers.

Additionally, nuts and seeds, such as almonds, walnuts, chia seeds, and hemp seeds, are excellent sources of protein and healthy fats. Whole grains like quinoa, amaranth, and brown rice also contribute to a well-rounded plant-based protein intake.

# Protein Supplements:

Protein supplements can serve as a convenient option for individuals who have increased protein requirements, such as athletes or those with certain health conditions.

Plant-based protein powders have gained popularity and are made from various sources such as pea, rice, hemp, and soy.

These powders can be easily incorporated into smoothies, shakes, or used in baking to boost protein content. It's important to note that while protein supplements can be a helpful tool, they should not replace whole foods in the diet.

Whole foods provide a wide array of essential nutrients, including fiber, vitamins, and minerals, that are often lacking in isolated supplements. Therefore, it is recommended to prioritize a balanced diet that includes a variety of whole plant-based protein sources alongside any supplementation.

Understanding the role of protein in supporting overall health and well-being is essential.

The best protein sources for healthy living encompass a variety of options, including both animal-based and plant-based sources.

By incorporating a combination of these sources into your diet, you can ensure a complete and balanced protein intake.

Whether you choose animal-based proteins like lean meats, poultry, and fish, or opt for plant-based proteins such as legumes, tofu, and nuts, the key is to prioritize quality and variety.

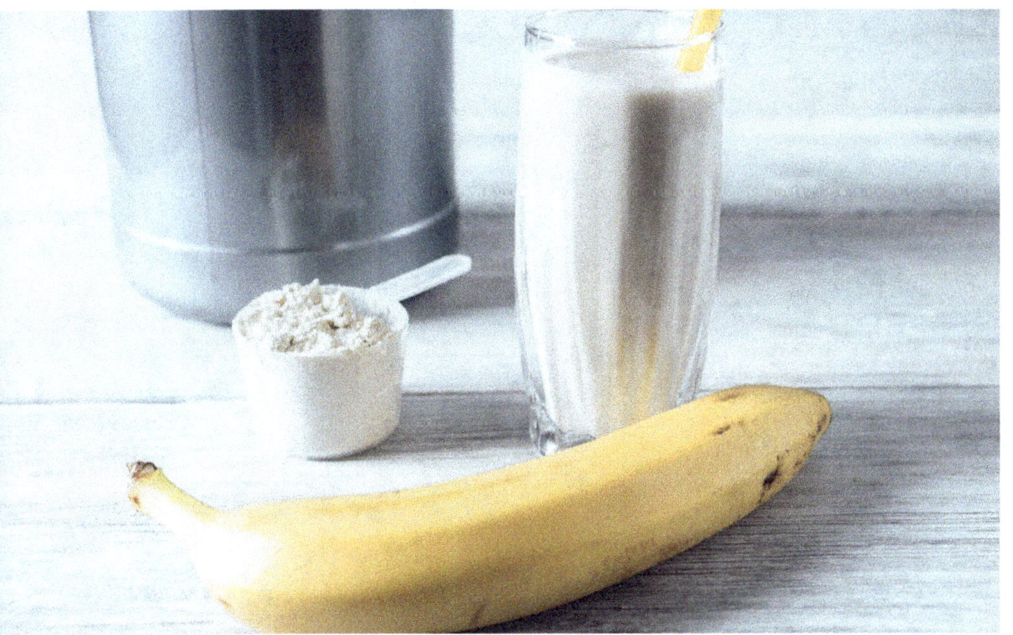

Additionally, considering individual needs and lifestyles, such as vegetarian or vegan preferences, can guide protein choices and ensure adequate intake.

By making protein a foundational component of your diet, you can support muscle development, promote satiety, and provide essential amino acids necessary for optimal health.


Remember, achieving a well-rounded protein intake is just one piece of the puzzle for overall health, and it's important to maintain a balanced and varied diet that includes other essential nutrients as well.

# Conclusion

In this short book I tried to create a comprehensive guide that delves into various aspects of nutrition and empowers readers to make informed choices for a healthier lifestyle.

Throughout the book, we explored the importance of a healthy diet as the foundation of overall well-being, understanding our relationship with food through mindful eating, and harnessing the healing power of food to optimize our health.

We talked about popular diet trends, shedding light on the truth behind them and helping readers navigate through the maze of information.

 We also highlighted the risks associated with processed foods and food additives, equipping readers with the knowledge to make conscious choices and prioritize their health.

The chapters on superfoods opened our eyes to the remarkable health benefits of fruits and vegetables, showcasing their rich nutritional profiles and their potential to support immune function, reduce inflammation, and promote heart and brain health.

We also explored the importance of incorporating the best protein sources into our diets to support muscle development, satiety, and overall vitality.

Throughout the book, we emphasized the importance of balance, moderation, and mindfulness in our eating habits. We encouraged readers to listen to their bodies, experiment with wholesome ingredients, and embrace sustainable and enjoyable eating patterns.

As you close this book, I invite you to embark on a lifelong journey of nourishing your body and mind through smart eating habits. Let this book serve as a guide, empowering you to make informed choices, discover the joy of wholesome foods, and prioritize your health and well-being.

Remember, small changes can yield significant results, and every step towards a healthier lifestyle is a step towards a brighter future.



Thank you for choosing "Smart Eating Habits"! May your journey towards optimal health be filled with vitality, happiness, and delicious nourishment.

To your health and well-being,

Steven Clinch

www.smarteatinghabits.com